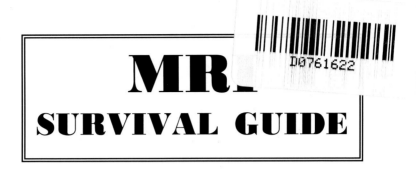

MRI
SURVIVAL GUIDE

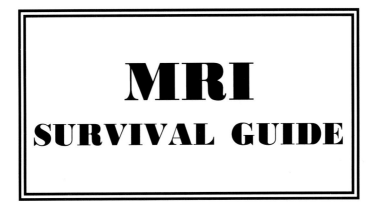

MRI
SURVIVAL GUIDE

JIM D. CARDOZA, M.D.
ALTA IMAGING MEDICAL GROUP
AND
MAGNETIC IMAGING AFFILIATES
BERKELEY, CALIFORNIA

ROBERT J. HERFKENS, M.D.
STANFORD UNIVERSITY MEDICAL CENTER
PALO ALTO, CALIFORNIA

RAVEN PRESS 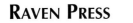 **NEW YORK**

Raven Press, Ltd., 1185 Avenue of the Americas, New York, New York 10036

Made in the United States of America

Library of Congress Cataloging-in-Publication Data

Cardoza, Jim D.
    MRI survival guide /Jim D. Cardoza, Robert J. Herfkens.
        p.   cm.
    Includes bibliographical references and index.
    ISBN 0-7817-0180-5
    1. Magnetic resonance imaging.   I. Herfkens, Robert J.   II. Title.
    [DNLM: 1. Magnetic Resonance Imaging.   WN 445 C268m   1994]
RC78.7.N83C37   1994
616.07'548—dc20
DNLM/DLC
for Library of Congress
                                                                            93-41765
                                                                            CIP

9   8   7   6   5   4   3   2   1

To Jennifer, Caitlin, Samuel, Tricia, Garrett and Meagan,
who were willing to share their husbands and fathers
with libraries and filerooms so that this book could be written.

Contents

Preface

This book provides the basic knowledge needed to begin interpreting MRI images. It is geared toward the practicing radiologist or radiology resident who has no formal training in MRI but is comfortable with cross-sectional anatomy and disease processes encountered on CT. This is a book that can be read in a single weekend and that will rapidly educate the reader to a level which will allow competent image interpretation. The radiologist can then use this body of knowledge to progress to standard texts and the imaging literature.

To achieve these goals, the physics of MRI is kept to a minimum. General concepts are presented that will be pertinent most of the time, without dwelling on occasional exceptions to the rules. Specific imaging sequences described are relevant to a G.E. Signa scanner but the general physical concepts are universal. The major and common disease processes of the CNS, body and musculoskeletal systems are presented along with imaging tips. There is no detailed discussion of pathologic processes, instead, characteristic MRI appearance will be presented to help in recognition and generation of a reasonable differential diagnosis.

It is hoped that readers will not feel intimidated by MRI. For many disease processes, the differential diagnosis is suggested by anatomic location, analogous to CT, albeit the anatomy is often better seen on MR. The signal characteristics can often reduce the process of differential diagnosis. We recommend that readers do not become discouraged or bogged-down in the "image construction and analysis" chapter. This material should be read quickly to get a feeling for the compromises that exist in image construction. Readers might then proceed to the clinical imaging chapters. Full understanding of the concepts presented in the image construction chapter is not strictly required when using established standard imaging protocols. As the reader gains experience, review of this chapter as well as familiarization with standard MRI texts is suggested. This will increase understanding of image acquisition as well as provide knowledge required for troubleshooting and image sequence design.

Acknowledgments

We would like to acknowledge the referring clinicians within the Alta Bates Hospital community of Berkeley, the Children's Hospital community of Oakland, and the Stanford University Medical Center community of Palo Alto, California. Their imaging referrals provided the case material in this book. Only physicians of the highest caliber and reputation could attract patients of such diverse pathology.

Thanks also go to Dr. Norbert Pelc for sharing his expertise of the physics of magnetic resonance, and to Peggy Cooley for her unwavering support and superb editing skills.

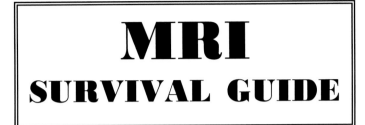

MRI
SURVIVAL GUIDE

1
Image Construction and Analysis

INTRODUCTION

This chapter is designed to provide a basic understanding of image acquisition and analysis. Some of the material that is presented here involves concepts derived from complex physics and mathematical functions. A simplification to the degree presented here mandates that generalities be made that may not be rigorously correct. They are correct to a sufficient degree to be useful to the practicing radiologist, allowing the construction and a reasonable interpretation of diagnostic images. Further reading of more rigorous texts is suggested after the basic concepts are understood and put into clinical use. In the beginning, it is suggested that the reader follow the established imaging protocols that are either set up by the manufacturer or, for readers operating a Signa system, those that are outlined in this book. As one gains expertise, changes in these parameters can be made to optimize a sequence for a particular clinical question. Before any changes in parameters are made, it is important to understand the consequences of each change in terms of the effect on the signal-to-noise ratio (SNR), spatial resolution, T1 or T2 weighting, imaging time, and the production of artifacts.

IMAGE ACQUISITION

A proton (i.e., the nucleus of hydrogen) has two physical properties that are important in magnetic resonance imaging (MRI). First, it has a net magnetic moment. As a result, if

placed in a magnetic field, it will tend to align with the external field. Second, it has angular momentum. This implies that, if it is not aligned with the external field, its magnetization will precess about the applied field, much like a spinning top that is not perfectly vertical in the earth's gravitational field. The frequency of precession is proportional to the strength of the applied magnetic field.

Images are acquired by placing the patient into a strong, homogeneous magnetic field. This tends to align the magnetic moment of a portion of protons within the patient's body with B_0, the external magnetic field (the z-axis), and establishes a net magnetization in the direction of the applied field ("longitudinal magnetization"). A radiofrequency (RF) pulse is applied at a frequency matching the proton's resonant spin frequency (the Larmor frequency). This pulse is of the correct intensity and duration to cause an effective 90° rotation of the magnetization into the xy-plane, resulting in the conversion of all longitudinal magnetization into "transverse magnetization." The transverse magnetization, as a result of being perpendicular to the applied field, precesses about it at the Larmor frequency, i.e., a frequency proportional to the strength of the applied field. This precessing magnetization can generate a measurable signal in a suitably arranged antenna (the receive coil). The return of the spins to the main magnetic field, when crossing the elements of an MRI antenna, induces a current and allows an RF signal to be

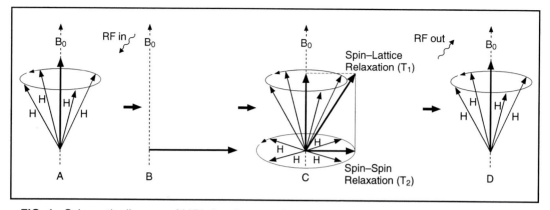

FIG. 1. Schematic diagram of MRI signal generation. **A:** The protons (*H*) align with and precess around the axis of the applied magnetic field (B_0), giving rise to a net spin vector along B_0 (*bold arrow*). **B:** An RF pulse is then applied which causes a 90° rotation in the net proton spin axis. **C:** After the RF is turned off, proton spin dispersion occurs in this new transverse plane (T2 relaxation), with re-aligning to the magnetic field (T1 relaxation). This change in the spin orientation causes an RF pulse to be transmitted from the patient. This is the means by which an image can be constructed. **D:** Given sufficient time, the proton spins become realigned to B_0.

detected (Fig. 1). It is from this RF signal that the MRI scan can be generated.

When the RF is turned off, two types of changes occur. The first results in a decrease in the net transverse magnetization. This is caused by slight differences in the precession rate of the protons that are the result of local inhomogeneity of the magnetic field (i.e., spin–spin relaxation). The decrease in the transverse magnetization is known as T2 relaxation or T2 decay. Second, the spins try to reach a lower energy state by realigning with the external magnetic field. The realignment of the spins with the external magnetic field and the reappearance of a magnetization vector aligned with the external field is known as spin–lattice relaxation or T1 relaxation (Fig. 1).

The actual location within the patient from which the RF signal was emitted is determined by superimposing magnetic field gradients on the otherwise homogeneous external magnetic field. For example, an x-directed magnetic field gradient, G_x, causes the magnetic field to vary linearly in the x direction. The applied gradient causes the Larmor frequency to depend on location in the direction of the gradient.

Localization in another direction can be achieved by applying a gradient along a second direction prior to signal read-out. This gradient causes a temporary frequency change and, therefore, a phase change, which is dependent on location in this second direction. Complete localization with this so-called "phase-encoding" method requires that the process be repeated multiple times, each with a different amplitude of the preparatory phase-encoding gradient, with the number of repeats being essentially equal to the number of desired resolution elements (pixels) in this direction. Together, frequency encoding and phase encoding generate a matrix of raw data, with the time interval along the read-out on one axis and the amplitude of the phase-encoding gradient on the other axis. A two-dimensional image can be produced by two-dimensional Fourier transformation.

Resolution in the third direction can be achieved by phase encoding also. This is used in three-dimensional imaging. More typical, however, is the use of selective excitation as a localization method in the third dimension. In selective excitation, the RF excitation pulse is applied in the presence of a gradient that causes the Larmor frequency to depend on position along the third direction. If the RF pulse contains energy only in a small band of frequencies, then MR excitation will occur only within the "slice" or "section" of the object within which the Larmor frequency matches the frequency content of the RF pulse. Slice thickness and location are controlled by the frequency content of the RF pulse and the strength of the gradient.

Along the frequency-encoding coordinate, 256 gradations generally are used in forming the image matrix. This can be increased without a significant scanning time penalty because all the frequency components are measured simultaneously during the read-out; however, this will have an impact on the SNR (discussed later). Unlike the frequency coordinate, increasing the number of resolution elements (pixels) in the phase-encoded direction incurs a time penalty because it requires a separate sequence repetition for each step. Increasing from 128 to 256 steps doubles the spatial resolution but also doubles the imaging time.

The SNR of the image depends linearly on the volume of the resolution element (voxel volume). The smaller the volume is (high spatial resolution), the lower the SNR is. It also depends inversely on the square root of the number of sequence repetitions and the length of time within each sequence during which the signal was acquired. Thus, halving the voxel volume in the slice in the frequency-encoded direction can be accomplished without increasing the scanning time, but this will halve the SNR. Halving the voxel volume in the phase-encoding direction might require a doubling of the scanning time to apply the necessary phase-encoding amplitudes. The voxel volume change causes the SNR to be halved, but there is an increase of the square root of 2 as a result of the scanning time increase, yielding a net SNR decrease of the square root of 2 (Fig. 2). Unique and innovative methods of sampling the acquisition data, such as fast spin–echo (FSE) or turbo acquisitions, allow much faster image acquisition.

To acquire all the data needed to produce an image, the pulse sequence is repeated a large number of times, generally between 128 and 1,024 times, to apply all the phase encodings and to perform the desired amount of signal averaging. The time that elapses from the 90°

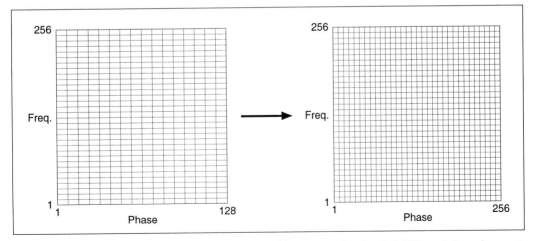

FIG. 2. Pixel matrix schematic. The frequency coordinate remains fixed at 256 gradations for most applications. The phase-encoded gradations can be varied. Increasing from 128 to 256 steps reduces pixel size (volume) by 50% and doubles the spatial resolution but reduces the SNR by one half. The scanning time also doubles because each phase-encoded step requires its own RF pulse for sampling. Because the sampling time is doubled, the SNR is increased by the square root of 2. This results in a net SNR loss by a factor of the square root of 2.

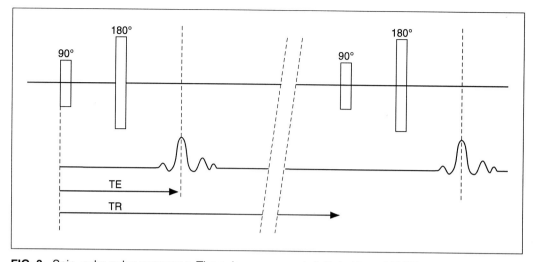

FIG. 3. Spin–echo pulse sequence. The pulse sequence is initiated by a 90° RF pulse. The TR represents the time that elapses from the beginning of one phase-encoded sampling to the beginning of the next (i.e., the time between the 90° RF pulses). The TE is the time the machine waits after the applied 90° RF pulse to receive the RF "echo" from the patient.

pulse of one repetition to the same pulse in the next repetition is termed the repetition time (TR). The time between the 90° pulse and reception of the MR signal emitted by the patient is termed the echo time (TE). The TR is longer than the TE, often much longer because of the need to control image contrast (discussed later). On standard spin–echo sequences, an additional RF pulse is applied at one-half TE to reverse any dephasing by 180° and maximize the MR signal (echo) at time TE (Fig. 3).

T1 AND T2 WEIGHTING

During the TE interval between the 90° pulse and signal reception, the transverse magnetization decays as a result of T2 relaxation; the shorter the T2 is, the lower the signal is. Because of technical constraints, it is impossible to make TE equal to zero. Lengthening the TE decreases the image signal but allows differentiation of tissues according to their T2 relaxation times. If TE is on the order of or longer than the T2 of some of the tissues, short T2 tissues will have lower signals than long T2 tissues because of their more rapid signal decay.

Another potentially significant tissue parameter is the proton density or the number of visible protons in each voxel. An image acquired with long TR and short TE is said to be spin density weighted or a proton density image because, while spin density will affect the image signal, T1 and T2 will not due to the long TR and short TE, respectively.

The selection of the TR and TE times determines if a sequence is "T1" or "T2" weighted. T1 weighting requires a short TR (> 800 msec, to allow differentiation according to T1) and a short TE (> 30 msec, to be relatively insensitive to T2 decay). The shorter the TR and TE are, the more T1 weighted the acquisition is. A T2-weighted sequence requires a long TR (< 2000 msec, to be insensitive to T1 differences) and a long TE (< 60 msec, to allow signal decay in short T2 tissues). A substance with a short T1 relaxation time has a high signal intensity (bright) on T1-weighted images because of its rapid recovery during the TR interval. Although all tissues will suffer some signal loss during the TE delay, a substance with a long T2 relaxation time is relatively bright on T2-weighted images as a result of the less rapid signal decay than occurs in short T2 tissues. A long T1 or short T2 relaxation time corresponds to low signal on T1- and T2-weighted images, respectively.

Generally, a diagnostic MRI examination contains a T1- and T2-weighted sequence in the same plane (usually axial) and a sequence (usually T1) in an orthogonal plane. Occasionally, additional special sequences are needed.

For the most part, the appearances of T1 and T2 weighting can be explained by the appearance of water and its local molecular environment and, to a lesser extent, by fat, because body tissues contain varying amounts of both. On a T1-weighted image, pure water is dark (low signal) and fat is bright (high signal intensity). On T2-weighted images, water is bright and fat is intermediate in signal intensity (it loses some signal intensity with respect to its appearance on T1-weighted images). Differences in the gray and white matter of the brain (as in the signal differences in other body organs) are in a large part caused by differences in water content. Fibrous tissue and cortical bone have a low water content and few free protons. This results in a low signal intensity, which appears dark on spin (proton) density and T1- and T2-weighted images.

The signal appearance of blood products on T1- and T2-weighted sequences is dependent on the oxidation state of hemoglobin. With age, hemorrhage progresses from oxyhemoglobin to deoxyhemoglobin to intracellular methemoglobin to extracellular methemoglobin (after red cell lysis occurs) and, then finally, to hemosiderin. Although the following rules hold more consistently in the central nervous system than the body, in general, deoxyhemoglobin is dark on T1 and T2. Intracellular methemoglobin is bright on T1 and dark on T2. After cell lysis occurs, the methemoglobin signal becomes bright on both T1 and T2. Further progression to hemosiderin causes a signal loss, becoming dark on both T1- and T2-weighted sequences (Table 1).

The intravenous contrast agent, gadolinium, shortens the tissue's T1 and T2 relaxation times. Its major effect, in appropriate concentration, is in T1 shortening, resulting in an increased signal on T1-weighted images. The clinical utility of gadolinium with MRI for the most part is similar to using iodinated contrast in computed tomography, but it carries with it less risk of allergic reaction and renal toxicity. Tissue with increased vascularity, such as neoplastic processes, tends to have an enhanced signal. Furthermore, gadolinium is bound to a large organic molecule which, under normal circumstances, is unable to cross the blood–brain barrier to enter the brain or spinal cord. When a focal breakdown in the blood–brain barrier is present, as occurs with a tumor or inflammation, gadolinium (like iodinated contrast) leaks into the region of abnormality, increasing its conspicuousness.

SPIN–ECHO SEQUENCES

The most commonly used sequence for diagnostic imaging is the spin–echo sequence. Standard T1- and T2-weighted images are spin–echo sequences. These sequences are obtained by adding an RF pulse of sufficient strength and duration to cause the proton spin axis to flip 180°. It is applied at a time which is one-half TE after the initial 90° pulse that initiates the TR (Fig. 3). This has the effect of reversing the protons' spin precession and refocuses the transverse magnetization at time, TE. This refocusing process results in two major advantages. The signal received is maximized, and heterogeneities of the static magnetic field are reduced. Both processes result in a better SNR. The major disadvantage of a spin–echo sequence is that it is costly in terms of imaging time, especially the T2-weighted

TABLE 1. *Signal intensity with T1 and T2 weighting*

Substance	T1	T2
Water	Dark	Bright
Fat	Bright	Intermediate to Bright
Cortical bone	Dark	Dark
Fibrous tissue	Dark	Dark
Deoxyhemo-globin	Intermediate to dark	Dark
Methemoglobin (intracellular)	Intermediate to Bright	Dark
Methemoglobin (extracellular)	Bright	Bright
Hemosiderin	Intermediate to dark	Dark
Gadolinium	Bright	Intermediate

sequences, because they require a long TR, which is a major determinant of imaging time.

FAST SPIN-ECHO (FSE) IMAGING

To reduce imaging time, particularly with T2-weighted sequences, and maintain the advantages of spin–echo imaging, an FSE sequence can be used. The actual acquisition of images with FSE is a complex process, but for this discussion, it is sufficient to say that the image time is decreased by acquiring multiple phase-encoding steps (instead of one) in each TR. The number of steps that are simultaneously acquired is called the "echo train" (ET). Typically, an ET of eight can be used. If all other parameters are held constant, this would reduce the imaging time by a factor of eight. However, to obtain an adequate number of slices, the TR often needs to be lengthened to approximately 4,000 (from 2,000 to 2,500). This increases the scanning time but also improves SNR and T2 weighting. The phase-encoding steps of the matrix can be increased to 192 or 256 (rather than 128), improving the image resolution. These changes result in a typical time reduction of approximately a factor of three to four over a standard spin–echo sequence. Note that the long TR requirements make FSE impractical for obtaining T1-weighted sequences in most applications.

Body imaging with FSE benefits from an increased number of excitations to average out respiratory motion and reduce the resultant artifact. However, several MRI body applications require actual calculations of T2 relaxation times. This can only be done with the standard spin–echo sequences. FSE should not be used in these calculations.

Another compromise of FSE imaging is its reduced sensitivity for the detection of blood products, particularly hemosiderin, compared with standard spin–echo sequences. Scans performed primarily to search for regions of hemorrhage, especially in the brain, should probably be done using a standard spin–echo sequence. Furthermore, myelination delay and dysmyelination in infants and children may be evaluated better with standard spin–echo sequences than with FSE.

GRADIENT-RECALLED ECHO (GRE) IMAGING

Other sequences have been devised to reduce the imaging time. Because these sequences do not use a spin–echo technique, the 180° refocusing RF pulse is not needed, allowing the TE to be markedly reduced (to as low as 2 to 4 msec). In turn, this also allows the TR to be reduced (to as low as 8 to 10 msec), markedly reducing the imaging time. A single-slice image can be obtained in as little as 500 msec. These GRE sequences offer major advantages and key disadvantages when compared with spin–echo sequences.

The tissue differentiation is poor because these sequences are neither truly T1 nor T2 weighted. Because of the extremely short TR, the protons do not completely relax between the sampling of the phase-encoding steps, resulting in residual transverse magnetization, which reduces the SNR. This is partially compensated by using an initial pulse that flips the proton's spin axis less than 90°, resulting in less residual transverse magnetization and improved SNR. There is an angle that optimizes the SNR (the Ernst angle). This is dependent on the prescribed TR and on the characteristics of the tissue being imaged. In the body, when a short TR (> 30 msec) is used, the optimal flip angle is approximately 30°.

In addition to SNR, there are other considerations in selecting the flip angle. The greater the flip angle is, the darker the appearance of water is. Conversely, smaller flip angles give water a bright appearance, resulting in a desirable myelographic effect in spinal imaging. Choosing a shorter flip angle can also result in optimal cartilage imaging, differentiating it from cortical bone and adjacent fluid. When the SNR becomes a problem and when flip angles other than the Ernst angle are needed for tissue differentiation, a multiplanar GRE sequence (MPGR) can be used. This sequence allows the simultaneous acquisition of multi-

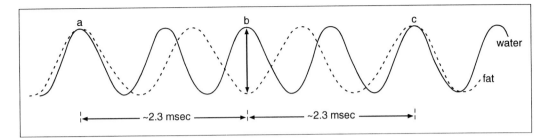

FIG. 4. The effect of TE on fat–water interfaces using nonspin–echo sequences. Representative sine waves are shown that demonstrate the concept of different characteristic frequencies (Larmor frequencies) of fat and water in a 1.5-T magnetic field. The signals are maximally additive at A and C, every 4.6 msec (1/220 Hz). They are maximally subtractive in the intervening 2.3-msec intervals (B). This phenomenon affects the appearance of the image at the fat–water interfaces. If the TE is chosen to put fat and water in phase, the maximal signal is created at the fat–water interfaces. Conversely, a TE chosen out of phase causes a minimal signal at the fat–water interfaces, giving sharply defined borders.

ple slices within a longer TR, rather than multiple single slices each with a shorter TR. The increase in TR results in an increase in SNR. An MPGR sequence is more motion sensitive than are single-slice acquisitions. This is because any brief movement degrades all simultaneously acquired slices, rather than just one slice, as occurs with single-slice acquisitions.

Another technique that can be used to increase tissue differentiation and SNR is a spoiled GRE sequence (SPGR). In this sequence, a complex RF pulse is applied to each TR to eliminate any residual transverse magnetization or T2 effects. These images have the appearance of T1 weighting and can be used to show the T1 effects of gadolinium enhancement. The SPGR sequence can also be obtained in a multiplanar (multiple slice) format (MSPGR).

Multiple factors enter into the consideration of the TE selection. Decreasing the TE to the minimal obtainable value results in increased SNR (the signal increases exponentially with decreasing TE) and, allowing maximum TR shortening, a decreased scanning time. However, with GRE sequences, optimal tissue contrast, i.e., fat and fluid differentiation, may not result. The spin frequency (Larmor frequency) of fat and water are different within the external magnetic field. At 1.5 T, this difference is approximately 220 Hz. This frequency difference causes the signal to be, alternatively, additive or subtractive at fat–water interfaces approximately every 2.3 msec (1/220 Hz). Choosing a TE value of approximately 2, 6, or 11 msec puts fat and water maximally in phase, giving the maximum signal to interfaces but blurring margins. With TE values of approximately 4, 8, and 13 msec, the fat and water signals are maximally out of phase, resulting in a decreased signal at the fat–water interfaces but causing sharp tissue margins (Fig. 4).

Often, GRE sequences are performed to evaluate the flow within blood vessels. With a short TE and single-slice acquisitions, flowing flood has a high signal intensity and appears bright. To enhance the vascular flow effects further, a flow compensation (FC) pulse (a gradient-moment nulling pulse) can be applied. This is not without price because it requires a longer minimum TE, creating the need for a longer TR and acquisition time. The FC involves a complex gradient that is added to the imaging sequence to normalize the signal from flow, either within a blood vessel or of the cerebrospinal fluid within the brain and spine. The flowing liquid becomes homogeneously bright. It is commonly used with standard spin–echo sequences to reduce the cerebrospinal fluid flow artifact in the cervical and thoracic spines.

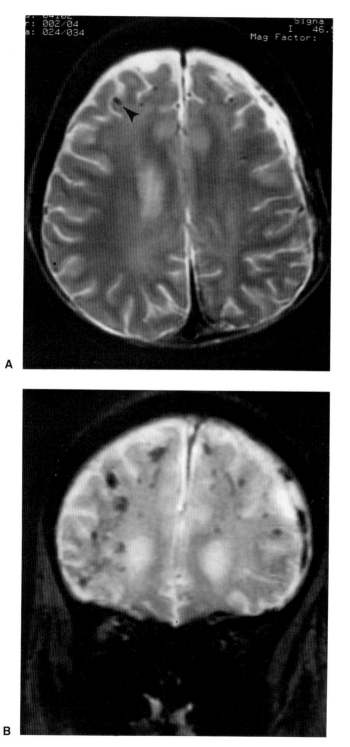

FIG. 5. Traumatic shear hemorrhages in the brain. **A**: The T2-weighted axial image demonstrates punctate low signal foci (*arrow*) at the gray–white junctions of the frontal lobes. **B**: A coronal MPGR sequence shows apparent enlargement or "blooming" of these foci because of a magnetic susceptibility artifact from hemosiderin deposition.

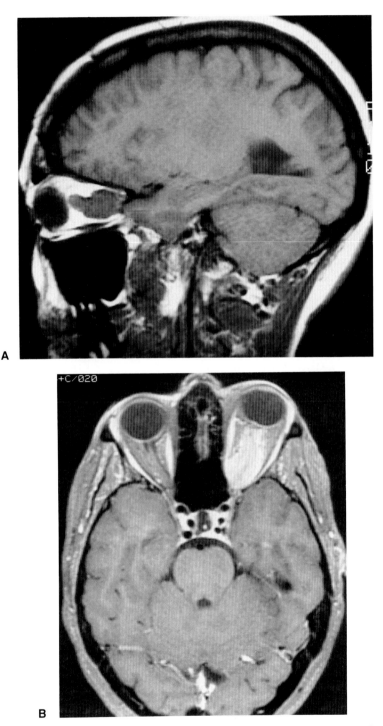

FIG. 6. Optic nerve meningioma. **A**: A sagittal T1-weighted image demonstrates an intermediate signal mass along the left optic nerve surrounded by high-signal-intensity orbital fat. **B**: An axial T1-weighted fat-sat image with gadolinium shows nulling of the signal from orbital fat, allowing easy visualization of the high signal tumor enhancement.

Because GRE sequences lack the refocusing 180° pulse present in the spin–echo sequences, they are more prone to include artifacts caused by local magnetic field inhomogeneities. This produces the "blooming" artifact that occurs in the presence of magnetic susceptibilities, such as calcification, iron-containing blood products, and air–water interfaces. Although these artifacts can obscure the anatomy, interfering with image interpretation, they can also be used to improve the image. A blooming artifact on a GRE sequence may be useful in confirming the presence of blood products, calcification, or air in a region of low signal intensity seen on a spin–echo T2-weighted sequence. These foci appear to increase in size (blooming) on a GRE sequence secondary to the magnetic susceptibility artifact (Fig. 5).

FAT NULLING SEQUENCES

Because fat and water have differing proton spin frequencies and T1 relaxation times, it is possible to design a spin–echo pulse sequence that nulls or saturates fat and preferentially displays water protons. These sequences are called fat saturation (fat-sat) or inversion recovery (STIR). Visually, these sequences markedly reduce the signal from fat, making it dark on the image. This is useful when evaluating the scan for a tumor or inflammation on T2-weighted sequences because these processes usually involve increased water content. Without a contribution of signal from fat, even subtle increases in water content result in easily visible signal. Fat-sat is also useful in orbital imaging. Using T1 fat-sat sequences to eliminate the signal of orbital fat, it is easy to evaluate for optic nerve pathological conditions by using gadolinium enhancement (Fig. 6). Without fat-sat, the bright signal from the adjacent orbital fat often obscures optic nerve or meningeal enhancement.

Like fat-sat, STIR imaging increases the sensitivity for detecting pathological increases in water content. Fat-sat is preferred by the authors because of the SNR, slice, and time penalty paid when using STIR sequences.

SNR CONSIDERATIONS

There is a a wide latitude in the ability to adjust MRI parameters. This allows the radiologist to design a study that answers specific diagnostic questions. Most adjustments made alter some combination of SNR, spatial resolution, image acquisition time, and the contrast-to-noise ratio.

The SNR is directly related to pixel volume (voxel size), whereas spatial resolution is inversely proportional to pixel volume. When all other parameters are held constant, if the matrix is altered by increasing the phase-encoding steps from 128 to 256, this halves the pixel volume, doubling the spatial resolution and imaging time. The overall effect on SNR is a reduction by the square root of 2 (because, even though the pixel volume is halved, the imaging time is doubled). Depending on other imaging parameters, this may result in a grainy image. Continuing with this example, to regain the previous SNR with the new 256 matrix, the number of excitations (NEX) required can be increased. The NEX is the number of times the entire sequence is scanned, allowing pixel averaging of the acquired data. However, SNR is not directly proportional to NEX, but rather to the square root of the NEX. Thus, the NEX would have to be increased by a factor of two to regain the square root of 2 loss in SNR. This increases the scan acquisition time by a factor of four (factor of two for the 256 matrix times two for the NEX) to maintain the same SNR.

Because the field of view (FOV) is two dimensional, SNR is proportional to the square of the FOV. For example, an FOV change from 28 cm to 14 cm, a factor of two, decreases the SNR by a factor of four (2^2) but also increases the spatial resolution by a factor of four (because two sides of the voxel have been halved). For smaller FOVs, the use of a smaller coil can dramatically increase the SNR without the need to increase the NEX and imaging time. In general, the smallest coil that will cover the region of interest and into which a patient will physically fit should be used.

A change in slice thickness also causes a corresponding change in the SNR. Reducing slice

TABLE 2. *Signal-to-noise dependence on imaging parameter changes*

Increasing image parameter	SNR
Matrix size	Proportional decrease[a]
Slice thickness	Proportional increase
FOV	Increases by the change squared
NEX	Increases by the square root of the change
TR	Exponentially increases
TE	Exponential decrease
Band width	Decreases by the square root of the change

[a]An increase in phase-encoding steps results in an overall square root SNR decrease because of the inherent proportionate increase in the imaging time.

thickness by 50% reduces the SNR by 50%, but spatial resolution increases by 50% (smaller voxel). Except for GRE and SPGR imaging (which are acquired one image at a time), slices in general on MRI should not be contiguous. To accomplish this, the sequence is prescribed with a slice thickness and an interslice gap. The gap is necessary to reduce "cross talk," which is essentially the effect of one slice on an adjacent slice. Cross talk information is a form of noise because it does not represent an anatomical signal pertinent to the specified slice. For body imaging in general (spin–echo imaging), to optimize the appearance of the image, it is best to have a gap between slices that approaches 50% of the slice thickness. This also has the advantage of increasing overall coverage of the body part with a limited number of slices allowed per TR.

Other major determinants of the SNR are the TR and TE. The SNR varies exponentially with these parameters. It increases with increasing TR and decreasing TE. For T2-weighted images, optimizing the TR and TE for SNR is difficult because a long TE is needed for T2 weighting, and although lengthening TR improves SNR, a significant time penalty is paid for the long TR. For T1-weighted sequences, shortening the TE as much as possible (with-

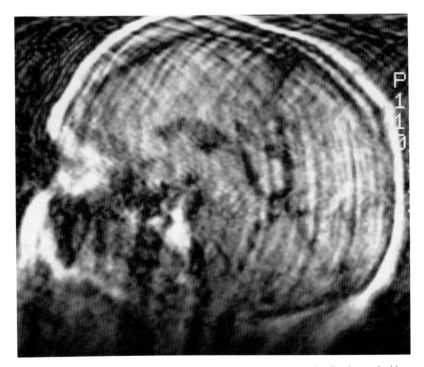

FIG. 7. Motion artifact. A T1-weighted sagittal image of the brain markedly degraded by motion during sequence acquisition.

out making it so short that the machine has only enough time to sample a fraction of the echo) creates a favorable situation on multiple fronts. It not only improves SNR, but also increases T1 weighting and the number of slices allowable per TR. An SNR penalty is paid for the short TR needed in T1-weighted imaging. However, the exponential gain in SNR by TE shortening usually more than compensates for this loss. For body imaging, it is suggested that the TR be set between 300 and 500 msec. This can be increased to 800 msec with neuroimaging because there are fewer tissue types needing T1 differentiation.

Changing the band width also affects the SNR. This will be discussed under the section on artifacts. Table 2 summarizes the SNR consequences of changes in imaging parameters.

ARTIFACTS

Artifacts are common in MRI scans. They can significantly degrade image quality and, at times, can confuse the imager by simulating a pathological condition. Examples of major artifacts will be demonstrated with brief descriptions to help in their recognition and, in some cases, their reduction or elimination.

Motion artifact is a major problem in MRI (Fig. 7). Unlike computed tomography, MRI usually acquires multiple images per sequence. If the patient moves at all during the sequence, not one, but all the slices in the region of motion will be degraded. It is important to make the patient as comfortable as possible during the scan to reduce the likelihood of motion. With difficult patients, it is sometimes wise to sacrifice spatial resolution, reducing the matrix size (e.g., from 256 to 128 matrix) to shorten the scanning time. A motion-free lower spatial resolution sequence may still be diagnostic, whereas a high-resolution scan with motion artifact wastes time and often is not diagnostic. With severe claustrophobia, premedication with benzodiazepines may be useful. Morphine or meperidine may also be helpful for pain control in patients who find it difficult to lie supine.

Respiratory motion is unavoidable in body imaging and adversely affects image quality. This artifact can at least be partially eliminated by attaching a respiratory bellows to the patient and using the machine software for respiratory compensation. This electronically rearranges the phase-encoding steps of image acquisition based on the patient's respiratory rhythm and the prescribed TR (this is called respiratory-ordered phase encoding). Using this technique, much of the respiratory "ghost" artifact is put out of the FOV, giving a crisper image (Fig. 8). Increasing NEX also reduces the artifact from respiration and from the random motion of bowel peristalsis by averaging out the motion on the image. For all abdominal imaging (chest, abdomen, and pelvis) when standard spin–echo sequences are utilized, respiratory compensation should be used.

Vascular pulsations are another form of unavoidable motion artifact. Similar to respiratory artifact, the vascular ghost from pulsations and blood flow occurs along the phase-encoding direction. Often, the velocity profile within the blood vessel itself is somewhat heterogeneous, with central flow being more rapid and coherent than flow near the vessel wall, which is slower and has higher velocity gradients. This can result in a heterogeneous signal profile within the vessel lumen. Much of this signal originates from adjacent slices in which the moving blood is experiencing the 90° RF pulse, but relaxation has occurred not in the slice excited but in a slice spatially removed. This flow artifact and vascular pulsatility artifact can be reduced by applying a presaturation pulse, spatially outside the specified slice, perpendicular to the direction of flow. This RF pulse eliminates the residual transverse magnetization, resulting in a signal void within the vessels (flow void, Fig. 8). Using an FC pulse also normalizes the intravascular signal, but, in this case, the flowing blood appears bright. Using either saturation or FC does have a time requirement and can reduce the number of slices per acquisition.

A chemical shift artifact occurs in the frequency-encoded direction. The magnitude of the shift artifact increases with increasing mag-

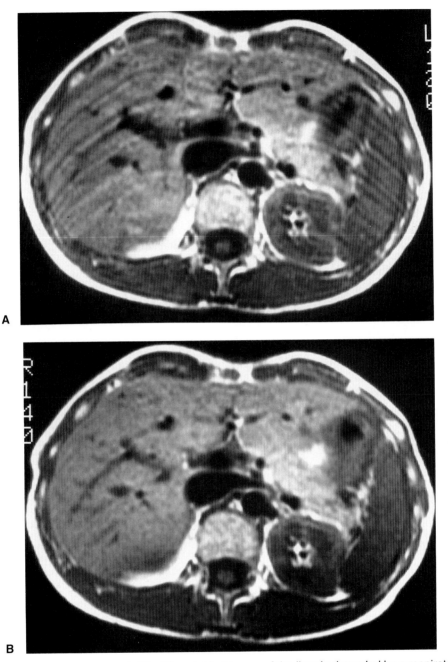

FIG. 8. Respiratory artifact. **A**: The T1-weighted image of the liver is degraded by a respiratory motion artifact. **B**: Holding all other parameters constant, the motion artifact is significantly reduced by the use of respiratory compensation. Notice that the application of a saturation pulse has eliminated the signal of flowing blood in the aorta and inferior vena cava.

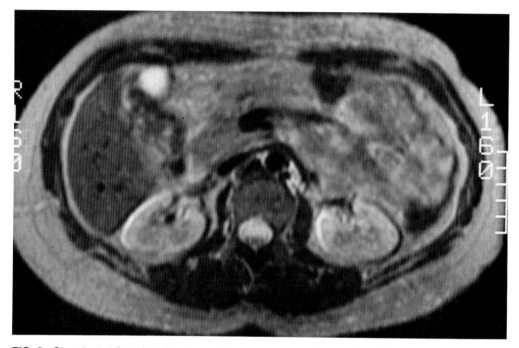

FIG. 9. Chemical shift artifact. The T2-weighted axial image through the kidneys demonstrate a bright band along the right and a dark band along the left (opposite) margin of each kidney. This 1.8-pixel shift is the result of a chemical shift at fat–fluid interfaces.

netic field strength. Fat and water have a 220-Hz difference in proton spin frequency (Larmor frequency) at 1.5 T. Spatial encoding in the frequency direction is performed by mapping the spatial position to frequency differences. Because fat and water have a 220-Hz difference in proton spin, there will be an apparent pixel shift of fat visualized at fat–water interfaces. This shift is approximately 1.8 pixels using a 256-pixel matrix, at a standard band width (16 kHz). Visually, the image shows a thin, bright band at one edge of a fat–fluid interface and a dark band at the edge on the opposite side (Fig. 9). Reduced band width is often used in neuroimaging to improve SNR. This is not a viable method for increasing SNR in routine body imaging, however, because of the abundance of fat–fluid interfaces. As the band width is reduced, the chemical shift artifact is increased (greater pixel shift) at these interfaces. This can obscure the margins of anatomical structures and pathological lesions.

"Wrap around" (aliasing) is an artifact that occurs when the body part being imaged is greater in diameter in the phase-encoding direction than the specified FOV (this can also happen in the frequency direction, but most current software packages compensate for this possibility). Anatomical areas outside the FOV are wrapped around and placed into the image (Fig. 10). This artifact is avoided by specifying an FOV greater than the patient's physical size, or by using the "no phase wrap" option (NP) when a smaller FOV is needed. With the NP option, the image is then acquired by doubling the number of phase-encoding steps and FOV in that direction and then discarding the added steps at the edges of the image. For example, a 128 matrix at two NEX is scanned as a 256 matrix at one NEX. Sixty-four phase-encoding steps on each side of the specified 128 steps are then essentially discarded. There is no cost in terms of time or SNR by using the NP option, even though the NEX is reduced by a factor of two. This is because the central

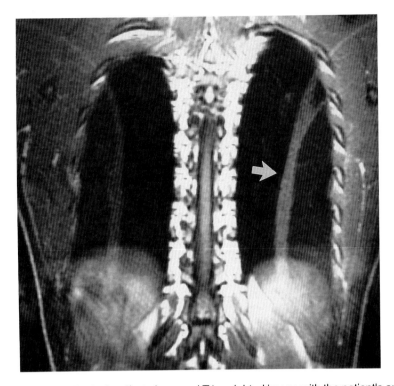

FIG. 10. A wrap-around (aliasing) artifact. A coronal T1-weighted image with the patient's arms (*arrow*) wrapped into the chest. The wrap-around artifact was created by failing to use the NP function while selecting an FOV in the phase-encoding direction that was smaller than the patient's anatomical size.

128 phase-encoding steps were actually sampled twice (256 matrix) because any time one phase-encoding step is sampled, sampling of all the steps mathematically occurs in the Fourier space (the mathematical means by which an image is generated from the scanning data). NP can be used with a one NEX acquisition but will result in a partial NEX sequence, which could degrade image quality.

Substances with weak magnetic properties (paramagnetic materials) cause magnetic susceptibility artifacts, resulting from alterations of the local magnetic field within the patient. This artifact is most prominent on nonspin–echo sequences, although it can also be seen on T2-weighted spin–echo images as regions of low signal (dark) at the foci of the paramagnetic material. On nonspin–echo sequences, these foci "bloom" or appear larger than their true size (Fig. 5). Ferromagnetic metals (iron, nickel, and cobalt) cause a marked distortion of the local magnetic field, resulting in signal dropout and the distortion of adjacent anatomy (Fig. 11).

Occasionally, a bright linear region of signal is seen centrally along the long axis of the spinal cord, which may mimic a syrinx. This is a truncation (Gibb's) artifact arising from insufficient sampling to define sharp borders in the mathematical process used in image reconstruction (Fourier analyses). This artifact can be reduced or eliminated by increasing the matrix size from 128 to 192, or preferably 256, phase-encoding steps.

SPECIAL IMAGING TIPS

As is true with essentially all examinations, with pediatric patients, it is important to

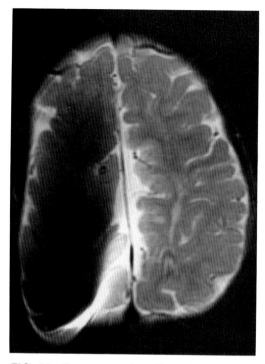

FIG. 11. Ferromagnetic artifact. An axial T2-weighted image shows distortion of brain anatomy as a result of a ferromagnetic artifact. The patient had a metallic shunt reservoir on the right.

use the smallest coil available that will cover the body part being scanned. For example, pediatric body imaging can often be performed in a head coil, markedly improving the SNR.

Motion artifact is the major culprit with pediatric patients. Nearly all patients younger than 6 years of age will require sedation. Although outpatient (out of hospital) sedation is relatively safe, sedation protocols should be developed with the referring pediatricians or pediatric anesthesiologists. Chloral hydrate or pentobarbital are effective agents.

The evaluation should be individualized. In general, patients with cardiac pacemakers, epicardial leads, central nervous system aneurysm clips (unless known to be made of tantalum), ear prostheses, or orbital metallic foreign bodies should not be scanned. Orbits can be screened for metal by a Caldwell view facial film or better with computed tomographic scanning, using 3-mm slices. The presence of a Starr-Edwards type of prosthetic heart valve with a metal ball in a metal cage is also a contraindication to MRI. The imaging of patients with all other major prosthetic heart valves is acceptable.

BIBLIOGRAPHY

1. Patz S. Basic physics of nuclear magnetic resonance. *Cardiovasc Intervent Radiol* 1986;8:225–237.
2. Gomori JM, Grossman RI, Goldberg HI, Zimmerman RA, Bilaniuk LT. Intracranial hematomas: imaging by high-field MR. *Radiology* 1985;157:87–93.
3. Yoshida K, Furuse M, Kaneoke Y, Saso K, Inao S, Motegi Y, Ichihara K, Izawa A. Assessment of T1 time course changes and tissue-blood ratios after Gd-DTPA administration in brain tumors. *Magn Reson Imaging* 1989;7:9–15.
4. Atlas SW, Grossman RI, Hackney DB, et al. Calcified intracranial lesions: detection with gradient-echo-acquisition rapid MR imaging. *AJR Am J Roentgenol* 1988;150:1383–1389.
5. Atlas SW, Mark AS, Fram EK, Grossman RI. Vascular intracranial lesions: applications of gradient-echo MR imaging. *Radiology* 1988;169:455–461.
6. Semelka RC, Chew W, Hricak H, Tomei E, Higgins CB. Fat-saturation MR imaging of the upper abdomen. *AJR Am J Roentgenol* 1990;155:1111–1116.
7. Wehrli FW, Perkins TG, Shimakawa A, Roberts F. Chemical shift-induced amplitude modulations in images obtained with gradient refocusing. *Magn Reson Imaging* 1987;5:157–158.
8. Tien RD, Hesselink JR, Szumowski J. MR fat suppression combined with Gd-DTPA enhancement in optic neuritis and perineuritis. *J Comput Assist Tomogr* 1991;15:223–227.
9. Kaufman L, Kramer DM, Crooks LE, Ortendahl DA. Measuring signal-to-noise ratios in MR imaging. *Radiology* 1989;173:265–267.
10. Wood ML, Runge VM, Henkelman RM. Overcoming motion in abdominal MR imaging. *AJR Am J Roentgenol* 1988;150:513–522.
11. Ehman RL, Felmlee JP. Flow artifact reduction in MRI: a review of the roles of gradient-moment nulling and spatial presaturation. *Magn Reson Med* 1990; 14:293–307.
12. Dwyer AJ, Knop RH, Hoult DI. Frequency shift artifacts in MR imaging. *J Comput Assist Tomogr* 1985;9:16–18.
13. Simon JH. Foster TH, Ketonen L, et al. Reduced-bandwidth MR imaging of the head at 1.5T. *Radiology* 1989;172:771–775.
14. Bronskill MJ, McVeigh ER, Kucherczyk W, Henkelman RM. Syrinx-like artifacts on MR images of the spinal cord. *Radiology* 1988;166:485–488.
15. Laakman RW, Kaufman B, Han JS, et al. MR imaging in patients with metallic implants. *Radiology* 1985; 157:711–714.

2

Brain

INTRODUCTION

Examination of the brain and spine with magnetic resonance imaging (MRI) has many distinct advantages over computed tomographic (CT) imaging. The "streak" artifact from bone that occurs with CT is absent with MRI. The multiplanar capabilities of MRI also allow better definition of pathological processes and their effects on adjacent structures. Greater differentiation of gray and white matter tracts is apparent, and often, the patency and course of intracranial vessels can be established without the use of an intravenous contrast agent. A key advantage of CT over MRI is its ability to detect accurately even small foci of calcification and acute hemorrhage.

Most examinations by MRI will involve an evaluation of both T1- and T2-weighted images. T1-weighted sequences best demonstrate anatomy (such as ventricular size and congenital malformations). T2-weighted sequences best demonstrate pathological conditions because most inflammatory and neoplastic processes appear bright in signal as a result of the increased water content.

A typical standard screening brain examination involves three sequences: sagittal T1 and axial T1- and T2-weighted images. Similar to CT, when reviewing MRI scans, it is best to establish a routine search pattern. This ensures that all major portions of the brain have been evaluated for pathological disorders. One such pattern for a standard brain study might proceed as follows (Fig. 1). Starting with the

midline sagittal, examine the corpus callosum, aqueduct of Sylvius, optic chiasm, hypothalamus, and pituitary gland. Next, check the clivus, sphenoid sinus, and pharyngeal tissues. In the posterior fossa, examine the brainstem, fourth ventricle, cerebellar vermis, and position of the cerebellar tonsils to exclude a Chiari malformation. Examine the cerebrum from left to right, also checking the orbits.

Next, moving to the T2-weighted axial sequence, check the orbits and sinuses. Starting at the foramen magnum, follow the brainstem to the thalamus, continuing cephalad to examine the basal ganglia region. Return to the posterior fossa, examining the cerebellum, fourth ventricle, and region of the internal auditory canals. Now, inspect the temporal, occipital, frontal, and parietal lobes from the base of the skull to the vertex. Notice the gray–white junctions, periventricular white matter, and the centrum semiovale. A similar but more cursory search is performed on the T1-weighted axial images, with particular emphasis on evaluating ventricular size and contour and sulcal size and looking for the presence of hemorrhage.

When a pathological process is encountered by MRI, it is usually detected by the presence of an abnormal signal and/or mass effect. If there is a focal space-occupying lesion, the multiplanar capability of MRI often helps to determine its position as intraaxial (within the brain parenchyma) or extraaxial (outside of the brain, distorting the brain's contour). This determination is key to the formulation of a differential diagnosis. In most cases, the location

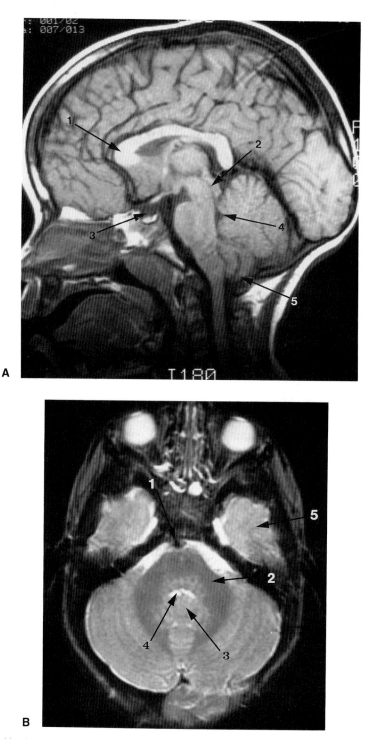

FIG. 1. Normal brain anatomy. **A:** A midline sagittal T1-weighted image demonstrates the corpus cal-losum (*1*), aqueduct of Sylvius (*2*), pituitary gland (*3*) in the sella turcica, the fourth ventricle (*4*), and the cerebellar tonsils (*5*). **B:** An axial T2-weighted image through the posterior fossa at the level of the pons demonstrates the basilar artery (*1*), middle cerebellar peduncles (*2*), vermis (*3*), fourth ven-tricle (*4*), and anterior temporal lobes (*5*, within the middle cranial fossa).

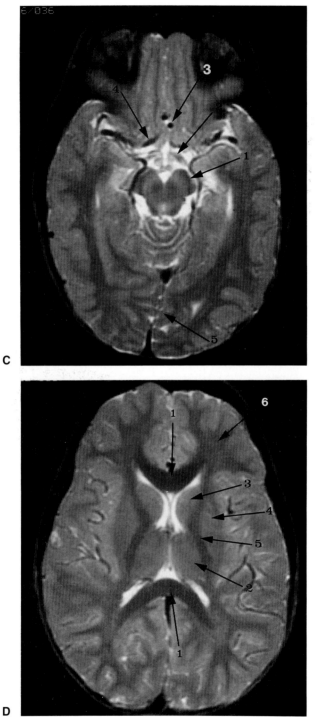

FIG. 1. *(contd.)* **C:** An axial T2-weighted image at the level of the midbrain demonstrates the cerebral peduncles (*1*), optic tracts at the chiasm (*2*), anterior cerebral arteries (*3*), middle cerebral arteries (*4*), and occipital lobes (with optic cortex, *5*). **D:** A T2-weighted axial image at the level of the lateral and third ventricles demonstrates the corpus callosum (*1*) with anterior rostrum and posterior splenium, the thalamus (*2*), the caudate (*3*) and lentiform nuclei (*4*), the internal capsule (*5*) with anterior and posterior limbs, and the frontal lobes (*6*).

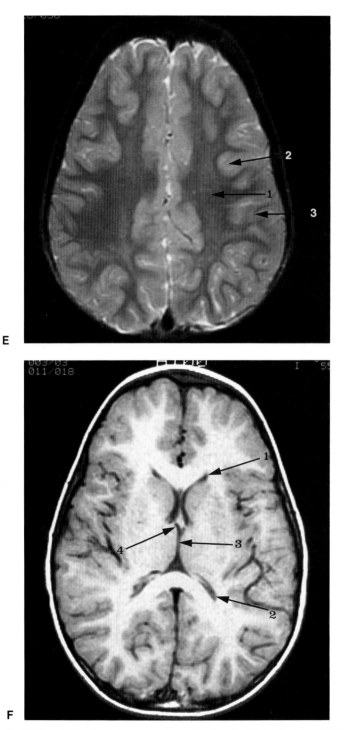

FIG.1. *(contd.)* **E:** A T2-weighted axial image above the level of the lateral ventricles demonstrates the low intensity white matter tracts of the centrum semiovale (*1*), the intermediate-signal cortical gray matter (*2*), and the parietal lobes (*3*). **F:** A T1-weighted axial image at the level of the lateral and third ventricles demonstrates normal-sized sulci and ventricles. The frontal horns (*1*) and atria (trigones, *2*) are demonstrated with the third ventricle (*3*), which communicates with the lateral ventricles through the foramina of Monro (*4*).

of the lesion and whether it is intra- or extraaxial is the most important factor to consider in terms of the differential diagnosis, although signal characteristics and enhancement patterns may shorten the diagnostic list of possibilities. In other words, the imager should not be intimidated by MRI because, similar to CT, the diagnosis is often suggested by the lesion's location. The real advantage of MRI over CT is its superior depiction of anatomy and increased sensitivity in the detection of lesions.

AGE-RELATED CHANGES

With age, brain atrophy occurs, which manifests as symmetric dilatation of the cerebral ventricles and sulci, best visualized on T1-weighted images (Fig. 2A). The concordant sulcal dilatation with the ventricular enlargement and lack of subependymal reabsorption of cerebrospinal fluid (CSF), i.e., a confluent increased juxtaventricular signal on T2-weighted sequences, help differentiate atrophy from hydrocephalus.

In addition to atrophy, punctate regions of increased signal intensity may be seen on T2-weighted images within white matter tracts that are a result of chronic small vessel ischemic disease (also called subacute atherosclerotic encephalopathy, SAE). These lesions can become more confluent, particularly in the periventricular white matter and centrum semiovale. Other locations also can be involved, including the brainstem, cerebellum, and basal ganglia (Fig. 2B,C).

The brain has a rich blood supply, and numerous small vessels penetrate and extend into the brain substance from the cortex. These blood vessels are invested in the meninges, forming perivascular spaces within which the CSF can track. At times, these perivascular spaces (Virchow-Robin spaces) are prominent and contain sufficient CSF to become visible as punctate foci of increased signal intensity within the white matter tracts on T2-weighted images. This normal variant, which may also be seen in younger patients, can often be differentiated from changes of chronic ischemia

by examining the first echo of the T2-weighted sequence (proton density images). The foci associated with perivascular spaces follow the signal of CSF, whereas the gliosis (scar) associated with changes of chronic ischemia are hyperintense to CSF on the proton density sequence (Fig. 3).

INFARCTION

The pattern of infarction on MRI is identical to the pattern on CT. If it is the result of a small vessel, such as a lenticulostriate or thalamoperforating artery, a lacunar infarct occurs (Fig. 4). Infarction from a major branch of a larger vessel, such as the middle cerebral artery, results in a wedge-shaped process extending to the cortical surface (Fig. 5A). Petechial hemorrhage, which presents as punctate foci of increased signal on the T1-weighted images, can be associated with infarction (Fig. 5B). It is seen more often on MRI than on CT. Unlike frank hemorrhage, this does not appear to be a contraindication to anticoagulation therapy.

In subacute infarction, the typical MRI appearance is an increased signal in the infarcted area on T2-weighted sequences, with a decreased T1-weighted signal. With time, the initial mass effect and edema resolve, and focal encephalomalacia persists. In the acute phase of infarction, vessels in the region of infarction may enhance with gadolinium secondary to a diminished intravascular flow (Fig. 6). The brain may otherwise appear normal.

HEMORRHAGE

Hemorrhage has multiple appearances on MRI, depending on its age (see Chapter 1). Most often, it will either be in the subacute phase (extracellular methemoglobin, bright on both T1- and T2-weighted images) or the chronic phase (hemosiderin, low signal, best seen on T2-weighted images). The signal characteristics help determine the chronicity of the bleed. Intracranial hemorrhage can result from a number of causes (Table 1). Similar to CT, the location of the blood, associated mass ef-

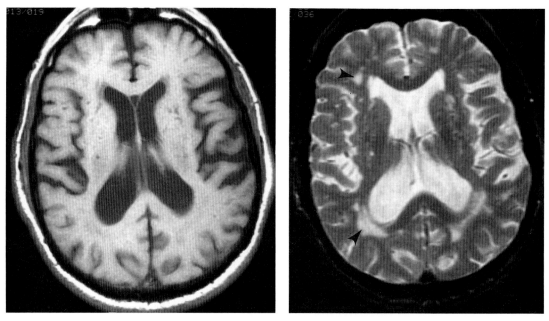

A

B

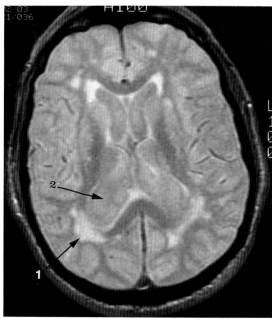

C

FIG. 2. Age-related changes in the brain of a 79-year-old patient. **A:** An axial T1-weighted image shows symmetric enlargement of the ventricles and sulci, indicating atrophy. **B:** The punctate and confluent regions of hyperintense signal, sometimes called UBOs (Unknown Bright Objects) in the periventricular white matter (*arrows*) seen on T2 weighting, result from chronic small vessel ischemic disease. **C:** Periventricular signal (*1*), which is hyperintense to the CSF (*2*), persists on the proton density image. This differentiates white matter pathological conditions from normal CSF in prominent perivascular spaces.

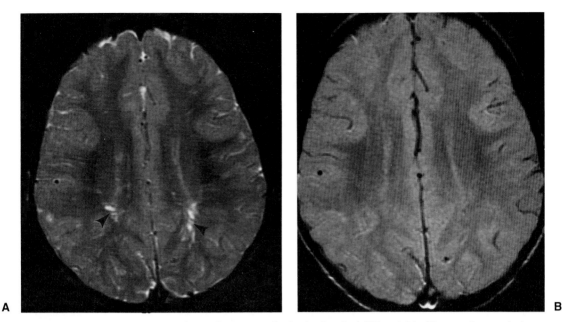

FIG. 3. Normal prominent perivascular spaces in the brain. **A:** A T2-weighted image demonstrates hyperintense signal in the posterior centrum semiovale (*arrows*). **B:** A proton density image at the same level fails to show hyperintensity but does shows a signal isointense with the CSF. This differentiates normal CSF-containing perivascular spaces from white matter disease.

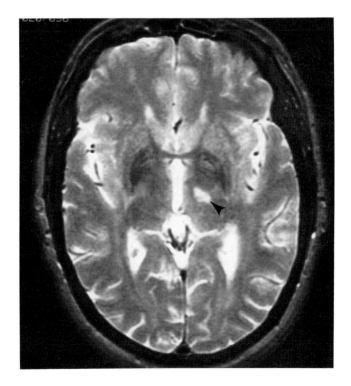

FIG. 4. Lacunar infarct. A T2-weighted axial image demonstrates a small hyperintense lesion without a mass effect in the left thalamus (*arrow*).

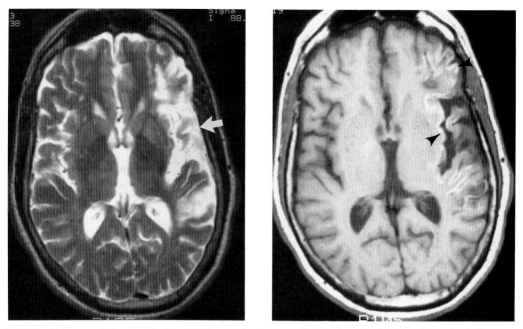

A   B

FIG. 5. Subacute infarction in the middle cerebral artery distribution. **A:** A T2-weighted axial image demonstrates hyperintensity in a large region of the infarction (encephalomalacia), extending to the cortical surface (*arrow*). **B:** A T1-weighted image at the same level reveals a rim of hyperintense signal at the cortical gray–white junction (*arrows*). This indicates petechial hemorrhage.

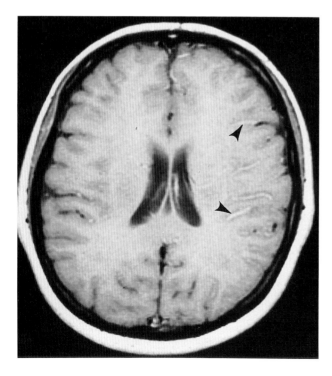

FIG. 6. Acute infarction. A T1-weighted axial image shows gadolinium enhancement of branch vessels in the left middle cerebral artery distribution (*arrows*). This indicates slow flow in the region of acute infarction.

TABLE 1. *Differential diagnosis of common sources of intracranial hemorrhage*

Vascular
    Aneurysm
    AVM
    Stroke
    Hypertension
    Neoplasm
Primary or metastases (especially renal,
    thyroid, and lung cancer; melanoma; and
    choriocarcinoma)
Trauma
Drugs (e.g., cocaine)
Infection (e.g., herpetic encephalitis)

---

fect, contrast enhancement pattern, and clinical history can go a long way in limiting the differential diagnosis.

Trauma can result in brain contusions and bleeding into the epidural, subdural, or subarachnoid spaces. In the acute setting, CT is the imaging modality of choice because it is more sensitive in the detection of acute hemorrhage (deoxyhemoglobin) and it tends to be more readily available. Furthermore, unlike MRI, life support equipment, such as a ventilator, can easily be used in the CT scanning suite. MRI is most useful in the subacute and chronic stages of hemorrhage.

The differentiation of a subdural hematoma (SDH) from an epidural hematoma (EDH) on MRI uses the same criteria as CT. An SDH forms a concave interface with the brain, and although it may be bilateral, it cannot cross the midline because its expansion is limited by the dural reflection at the falx. An EDH, on the other hand, forms a convex interface with the brain and may cross the midline (Fig. 7). Both SDH and EDH are serious conditions as a result of the mass effect exerted on the adjacent brain, which may result in a brain herniation. An EDH generally results from an arterial bleed and tends to progress rapidly. An SDH generally results from a venous bleed, and although rapid progression may occur, it can be indolent.

In severe trauma, occasionally, a rotatory force is present in which the gray matter and white matter rotate at slightly different rates because of their differences in specific gravity. When this occurs, tiny shear hemorrhages at these gray–white interfaces and within the corpus callosum occur. The presence of shear hemorrhages is a poor prognostic sign. Detection of this abnormality is optimized by using a gradient-recalled echo (GRE) technique, such as multiplanar GRE, which allows "blooming" of the blood products (see Chapter 1, Fig. 5).

Hypertensive bleeds commonly occur in the basal ganglia, but they may involve the internal capsule, thalamus, brainstem, or cerebellum. They are intraaxial and are associated with edema acutely. As the high signal on T1-weighted images from methemoglobin resolves, a follow-up scan with gadolinium is indicated to exclude a neoplasm as a possible source of hemorrhage.

VASCULAR ABNORMALITIES

Cerebral aneurysms may present clinically with bleeding into the subarachnoid space, causing a severe headache, or may be incidentally found on a CT or MRI scan. Aneurysms most commonly arise from the circle of Willis and occur in the following locations at descending frequency: anterior communicating artery, trifurcation of the middle cerebral artery, posterior cerebral artery, basilar tip, and posterior inferior cerebellar artery. They are multiple in up to 20% of cases. Typically, on MRI, they present as a focal rounded extension of a vascular structure. If thrombosed or partially thrombosed, a laminated appearance of differing signal intensity may be present along the aneurysmal wall, resulting from a thrombus of varying ages. A GRE (flow-sensitive) sequence is useful in defining blood flow within the aneurysm (Fig. 8).

A good way to screen for intracranial aneurysms or vascular malformations, short of conventional angiography, is with MR angiography (MRA). A three-dimensional time-of-flight technique gives good visualization of the vessels in the circle of Willis under most circumstances. A macroscopic aneurysm with

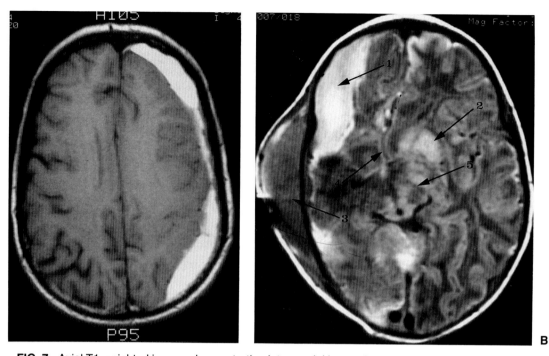

FIG. 7. Axial T1-weighted images demonstrating intracranial hemorrhage as a result of child abuse. **A:** A 3-year-old child with a hyperintense SDH on the left. Notice the concave interface with the brain and the associated mass effect evidenced by ipsilateral sulcal effacement. **B:** Postoperative study of a 5-month-old child with a right frontal epidural hematoma (*1*), forming a convex interface with the brain. Intraparenchymal hemorrhage (*2*) and scalp hematoma (*3*) are also present. The mass effect causes subfalcine herniation (midline shift, *4*), uncal herniation with brainstem rotation (*5*), and sulcal effacement on the right.

flow present can be identified. This provides projections similar to conventional angiography, showing the vascular anatomy in the anteroposterior, lateral, and oblique projections (Fig. 9). Also, MRA can be used to screen for arteriovenous malformations (AVM) and atherosclerotic disease of the carotid arteries. When a hemorrhage or thrombus is present, the bright signal can obscure the vascular anatomy on three-dimensional time-of-flight sequences because of their relative T1 weighting. Under these circumstances, phase-contrast MRA may be most useful.

Vascular malformations include capillary telangiectasias, venous angiomas, and AVMs. Venous angiomas are generally silent clinically. MRI may demonstrate a spoked-wheel pattern of small vessels (veins), which appear situated within the brain parenchyma (Fig. 10).

Capillary telangiectasias and occult AVMs are detected only by imaging studies if hemorrhage occurs. These lesions then manifest focal, intraparenchymal hemorrhage of differing ages, giving a laminated appearance. Associated vessels are usually not present (Fig. 11). Edema is also typically absent, except after an acute bleed. Careful evaluation is warranted to exclude a hemorrhagic neoplasm.

Large AVMs typically present as a tangle of vessels with a large abnormal draining vein. Unless hemorrhage is present, little or no mass effect is seen. Most are supratentorial. An intravascular flow void is seen on spin–echo images (Fig. 12). In addition, GRE (flow-sensitive) images may be useful to define the vascular anatomy further.

Venous thrombosis can also be diagnosed by MRI. A thrombus can be visualized that oc-

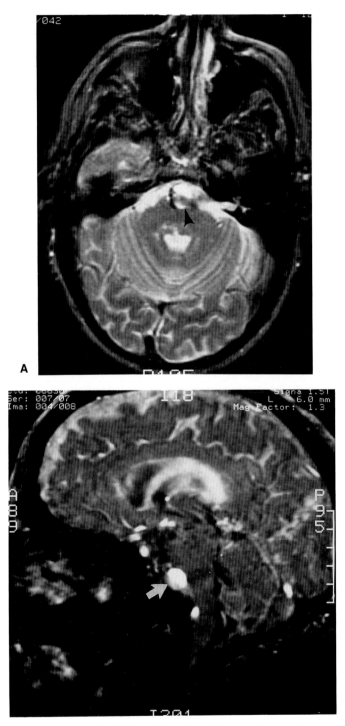

FIG. 8. Basilar artery aneurysm. **A:** A T2-weighted axial image demonstrates a rounded 1.5-cm aneurysm arising from the basilar artery (*arrow*). **B:** The GRE sagittal image demonstrates blood flow, which is bright, and a thrombus, which is intermediate in signal (*arrow*), within the aneurysm.

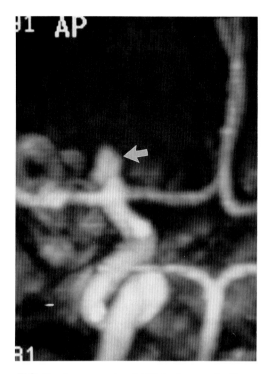

FIG. 9. An example of MRA, demonstrating a middle cerebral artery aneurysm (*arrow*).

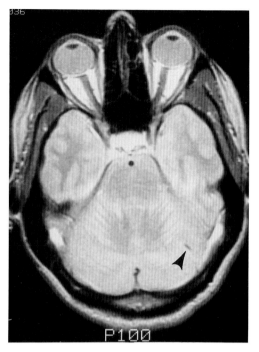

FIG. 10. Venous angioma. Proton density image demonstrating an aberrant vessel in the left cerebellar hemisphere draining centrally. A spoked-wheel pattern is not seen.

cludes the superior sagittal or other major sinus. The lack of flow can be further confirmed with a GRE (flow-sensitive) sequence. Venous occlusion can result in infarction of the brain in a distribution that corresponds with venous drainage rather than the more typical distribution of arterial supply. These infarcts are often hemorrhagic (Fig. 13).

INFECTION

Bacterial cerebritis or meningitis can result from the direct spread of bacteria from an ear, nose, or throat source or by hematogenous spread of an extracranial infection. In the case of cerebritis, the hematogenously acquired lesions are usually located at the gray–white junction and may be solitary or multiple. Regions of cerebritis typically have an increased T2-weighted signal, with the signal slightly hypointense to the signal in the adjacent brain on T1-weighted images. A mass effect is present with effacement of sulci and, sometimes, the ventricles. Hemorrhage may be present (bright on T1).

Cerebritis can be treated medically. With further progression, central necrosis occurs, and an abscess forms. An abscess typically is surrounded by gliosis (scar). The gliotic capsule tends to be mildly hyperintense on T1-weighted sequences and mildly hypointense on T2-weighted sequences compared with the adjacent brain. Gadolinium produces capsular enhancement, which typically is relatively smooth and thin. This is variable, however. A large amount of edema, typically following white matter tracts (vasogenic edema), is usually present, contributing to the mass effect (Fig. 14). The major differential diagnostic considerations for a ring-enhancing lesion in the brain are listed in Table 2.

When meningitis is present, often the precontrast MRI scans are normal; however, as in

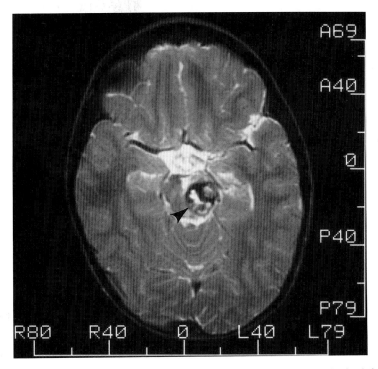

FIG. 11. Cryptic AVM. A T2-weighted axial image demonstrates hemorrhage in the left cerebral peduncle *(arrow)*. Abnormal vessels are typically not seen. The heterogeneous, laminated regions of differing signal result from differing oxidation states of the hemorrhagic products.

contrast-enhanced CT, T1-weighted post-gadolinium MRI scans may demonstrate increased meningeal enhancement (Fig. 15). The inflamed meninges can cause spasm or thrombosis in adjacent vessels, resulting in infarction, or they can cause cerebritis in the adjacent brain. Tuberculus meningitis is the prototype for these complications. Further complications include extraaxial empyemas and hydrocephalus.

TABLE 2. *Differential diagnosis of ring-enhancing brain lesions*

Astrocytoma
Metastasis
Infarction (including vasculitis)
Abscess (including toxoplasmosis)
AVM
Demyelination
CNS lymphoma (AIDS)

The appearance of fungal meningitis with its complications are indistinguishable from tuberculosis, either on MRI or CT. The imaging modality of choice is MRI because of reduced artifact at the base of the skull, a preferred site for infection by tuberculosis or fungi. It is rare to have brain parenchymal involvement when fungal meningitis is present, but enhancing granulomas or abscesses can occur. In general, MRI (or CT) cannot determine which particular fungus is the infecting agent. In patients with acquired immunodeficiency syndrome (AIDS), however, cryptococci have been shown to cause nonenhancing enlargement of perivascular spaces in the basal ganglia and midbrain (Fig. 16). These correspond pathologically to fungus-filled Virchow-Robin spaces.

Patients with AIDS and other immunocompromised patients are also susceptible to parasitic infections, particularly toxoplasmosis.

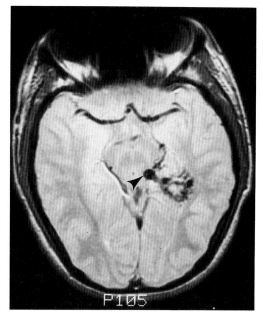

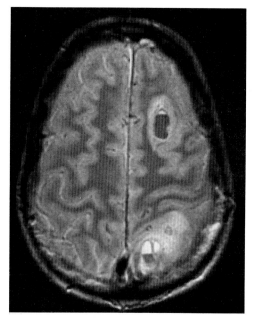

FIG. 12. Large AVM. The proton density axial image demonstrates a tangle of large vessels in the medial left temporal lobe draining into a large vein (*arrow*) within the perimesencephalic cistern.

FIG. 13. Venous infarction. A T2-weighted axial image in a patient with a superior sagittal sinus thrombosis demonstrates multiple hemorrhagic infarcts. Notice that the areas of infarction do not follow a typical arterial distribution.

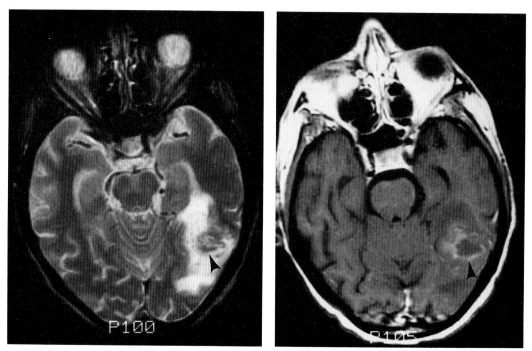

A

B

FIG. 14. Cerebritis forming an abscess. **A:** A T2-weighted image shows findings of cerebritis with early abscess formation in the posterior left temporal lobe (*arrow*). Note the large amount of surrounding high signal edema following the white matter tracts. **B:** A T1-weighted axial image with gadolinium demonstrates thin capsular enhancement (*arrow*).

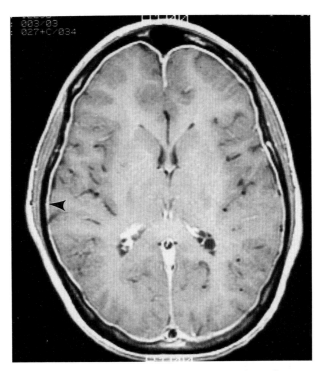

FIG. 15. Viral meningitis. A T1-weighted image with gadolinium shows intense meningeal enhancement (*arrow*).

This opportunistic organism can occur anywhere but favors the basal ganglia and gray–white junctions. The lesions are often hyperintense on T2-weighted sequences, but they are variable and may be isointense with surrounding brain. A mass effect and edema are typically present with ring enhancement using gadolinium on T1-weighted sequences (Fig. 17). Hemorrhage within the lesions is sometimes seen. When ring-enhancing lesions are found in the setting of AIDS, empirical antibiotic treatment for toxoplasmosis is initiated. A decrease in the size of the lesion and edema is expected within several weeks. If unresponsive, lymphoma should be considered.

Congenital toxoplasmosis results during pregnancy when the parasite crosses the placenta to infect the developing fetus. Similar to other TORCH infections (rubella, cytomegalovirus, and herpes), encephalitis with brain destruction, atrophy, and hydrocephalus can occur. The structural and clinical severity depends on the gestational age at the time of infection.

Cysticercosis is caused by the pork tapeworm, *Taenia solium*. When central nervous system (CNS) involvement occurs, it is generally parenchymal, but the cerebral ventricles (and CSF spaces) and meninges can also be involved. The symptoms generally are seizures from parenchymal involvement or hydrocephalus from intraventricular involvement.

Parenchymal lesions usually occur at the cerebral gray–white junctions. Early in the infection, a small enhancing nodule can be seen with focal edema. This progresses to a ring-enhancing lesion, usually 1 to 2 cm in size (Fig. 18). The lesion eventually regresses (within 5 years if untreated), and focal calcification may persist. Although MRI is superior in detecting parenchymal lesions and intraventricular cysts, the calcified focus is better detected by CT.

Although viral encephalitis and/or meningitis may be caused by one of many viruses, probably the more common are Coxsackie, human immunodeficiency (HIV), herpes simplex, and papovaviruses (progressive multifo-

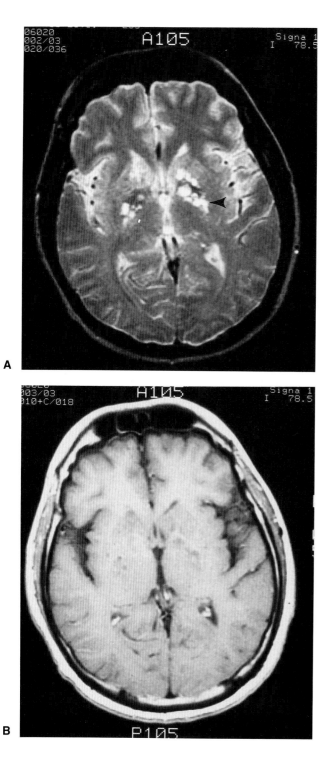

A

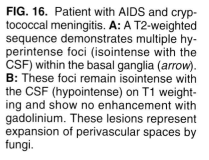

FIG. 16. Patient with AIDS and cryptococcal meningitis. **A:** A T2-weighted sequence demonstrates multiple hyperintense foci (isointense with the CSF) within the basal ganglia (*arrow*). **B:** These foci remain isointense with the CSF (hypointense) on T1 weighting and show no enhancement with gadolinium. These lesions represent expansion of perivascular spaces by fungi.

B

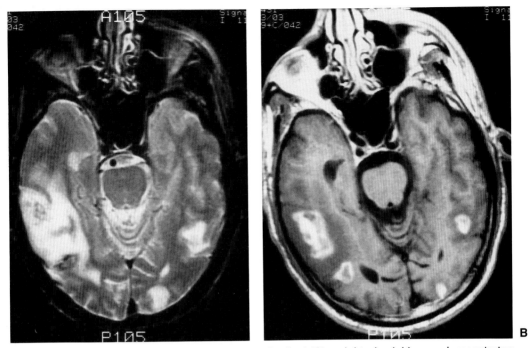

FIG. 17. Patient with AIDS and CNS toxoplasmosis. **A:** A T2-weighted axial image demonstrates multiple hyperintense lesions or edema at the gray–white junctions. **B:** A T1-weighted image with gadolinium demonstrates multiple ring-enhancing lesions with surrounding low-signal edema.

TABLE 3. *Myelination changes with age*

Anatomic region	T1 weighting	T2 weighting
Middle cerebellar peduncle	Birth	Birth–2 mo.
Cerebellar white matter	Birth–4 mo.	3–5 mo.
Posterior limb internal capsule		
Anterior portion	Birth	4–7 mo.
Posterior portion	Birth	Birth–2 mo.
Anterior limb internal capsule	2–3 mo.	7–11 mo.
Genu corpus callosum	4–6 mo.	5–8 mo.
Splenium corpus callosum	3–4 mo.	4–6 mo.
Occipital white matter		
Central	3–5 mo.	9–14 mo.
Peripheral	4–7 mo.	11–15 mo.
Frontal white matter		
Central	3–5 mo.	9–14 mo.
Peripheral	7–11 mo.	14–18 mo.
Centrum semiovale	2–4 mo.	7–11 mo.

Adapted from Barkovich et al. *Radiology* 1988; 166:173–180, with permission.

cal leukoencephalopathy, PML). They all have a predilection for white matter involvement and tend to be multifocal to diffuse in distribution. Typically, these lesions are bright on T2-weighted sequences and isointense or hypointense to normal brain on T1-weighted sequences. It is difficult to determine the actual infecting agent accurately by imaging characteristics alone. However, combining the imaging characteristics with the patient's clinical history can be useful in suggesting a likely differential diagnosis. Because of its improved sensitivity over CT in detecting white-matter changes, MRI is the imaging modality of choice.

In acute viral encephalitis, cerebral edema typically occurs, causing a mass effect and effacing sulci. Breakdown of the blood–brain barrier can be detected by gadolinium enhancement on T1-weighted images. Meningeal enhancement suggests associated meningitis.

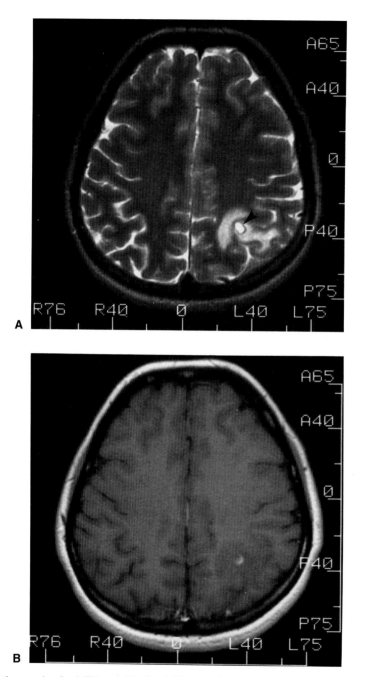

FIG. 18. Cysticercosis. **A:** A T2-weighted axial image demonstrates a small hyperintense nodule (*arrow*) with surrounding edema at the gray–white junction. **B:** A T1-weighted image with gadolinium shows enhancement of the cysticercosis nodule.

In chronic encephalitis, atrophy is present instead of a mass effect.

Herpetic encephalitis is often unilateral and has a predilection for the temporal and inferior frontal lobes. It often spares the adjacent putamen (Fig. 19). A mass effect is typical. Hemorrhage into the affected brain may be present.

Unlike herpetic or other acute viral encephalitides, the changes seen with HIV infection are atrophy rather than a mass effect. Typically, the atrophic changes begin in the subcortical white matter and then become generalized, causing enlargement of the sulci and ventricles. High-signal-intensity lesions on T2-weighted images develop in the periventricular white matter and centrum semiovale. These lesions represent demyelination and tend to become confluent. No mass effect or gadolinium enhancement is typically seen.

It is often difficult to differentiate the changes of HIV infection from those of PML (papovavirus, which occurs in approximately 4% of patients with AIDS). These lesions can occur anywhere in the brain but tend to be asymmetrical with a predilection for the subcortical white matter (Fig. 20), especially in the centrum semiovale posteriorly. Small lesions become confluent as the infection progresses. Death from PML usually occurs within 6 months.

WHITE MATTER DISEASES

To recognize pathological conditions involving the white matter tracts of the brain, it first is important to recognize the normal white matter appearance because this appearance changes with age. These changes are best seen with MRI. Myelination begins *in utero* and continues after birth. In general, it progresses from caudal to cephalad and dorsal to ventral. Sensory pathways tend to myelinate before motor pathways. On T1-weighted images, the white matter tracts progress from hypointense to hyperintense (compared with gray matter) as myelination occurs. This signal change is reversed on T2-weighted sequences. The changes of myelination in general are seen earlier on

T1- and later on T2-weighted sequences (Fig. 21). By 2 years of age, the myelination pattern should be the adult form. The MRI myelination milestones (Table 3) should be checked when imaging infants to determine whether a myelination delay is present. When imaging children younger than 2 years of age, the degree of myelination is better seen when the T2-weighted sequence uses a prolonged TE (i.e., 100 to 120 msec).

During the perinatal period, the watershed areas are in the periventricular regions. An ischemic event in this period results in periventricular leukomalacia. This is usually found in the periatrial white matter and results in thinned white matter tracts and a persistently increased white matter signal on T2-weighted images after myelination is complete (Fig. 22). Associated thinning of the posterior body of the corpus callosum may also be present.

Multiple sclerosis is a relatively common demyelinating disorder that can cause visual impairment, weakness, numbness, and gait disturbance. The diagnosis is based on clinical criteria, which include evidence of at least two spatially separate lesions in the CNS; MRI is superior to CT in detecting these lesions. Acutely, active regions of demyelination are hyperintense to the surrounding brain on T2-weighted images. The lesions enhance with gadolinium on T1-weighted sequences and may have a focal mass effect. Chronically, after active demyelination has stopped, the lesion (plaque) retains its bright signal on T2 but no longer enhances with gadolinium. With increase in lesion size and number, atrophy becomes apparent. Imaging during symptom exacerbation can find coexistent enhancing foci of acute demyelination with chronic inactive plaques (Fig. 23).

The demyelinating plaques of multiple sclerosis can occur anywhere within the brain and spinal cord, but usually, they involve white matter tracts and favor the periventricular regions. Morphologically, these plaques may be difficult to distinguish from changes of chronic ischemia, and although 90% of patients with multiple sclerosis present before 50 years of age, some overlap occurs in which age-relat-

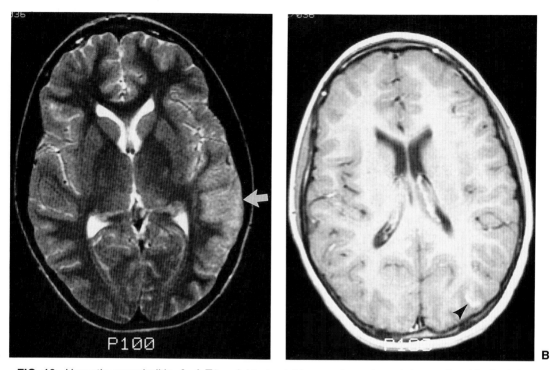

FIG. 19. Herpetic encephalitis. **A:** A T2-weighted axial image shows hyperintense signal in the left temporal lobe (*arrow*). **B:** A small amount of gyral enhancement was seen posteriorly on T1 weighting with gadolinium (*arrow*).

ed white matter ischemic changes are expected. A sagittal T2-weighted sequence may help in differentiating between the plaques of multiple sclerosis and ischemic lesions because the former commonly involve the corpus callosum, especially the undersurface of the callosal body (Fig. 24). Ischemic changes in this region are rare.

Radiation and chemotherapy can also cause white matter abnormalities. Some changes are transient, but some are permanent and can be associated with severe neurological deficits. Edema with a hyperintense signal in deep white matter tracts can occur with either radiation therapy (vasculitis), high-dose intravenous methotrexate, or combination drug therapy (Fig. 25). Multifocal white matter necrosis and resultant atrophy follows if permanent damage occurs. Permanent damage is unusual following chemotherapy.

In addition to demyelinating disorders, multiple dysmyelinating processes have also been described involving inborn errors in synthesis or metabolism. These conditions are rare and, with few exceptions, cause nonspecific changes in the white matter tracts.

TUMORS

For the evaluation of most brain tumors, MRI is the method of choice. As mentioned previ-

TABLE 4. *Major intraaxial hemispheric neo-plasms*

Astrocytoma
Glioblastoma multiforme
JPA
Oligodendroglioma
PNET
Hemangioblastoma
Metastasis
Lymphoma (primary)

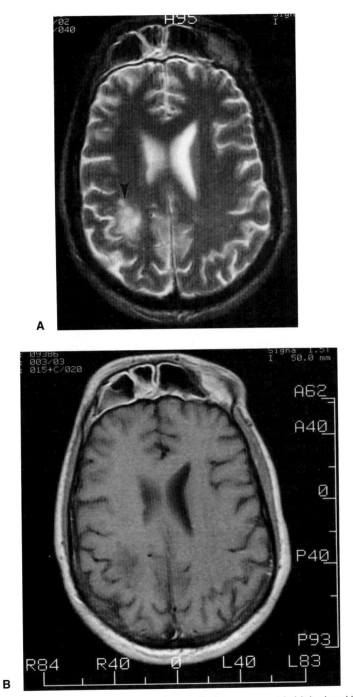

FIG. 20. PML. **A:** A T2-weighted axial image demonstrates asymmetric high signal lesion in the posterior subcortical white matter on the right (*arrow*). **B:** A T1-weighted image with gadolinium shows no lesion enhancement.

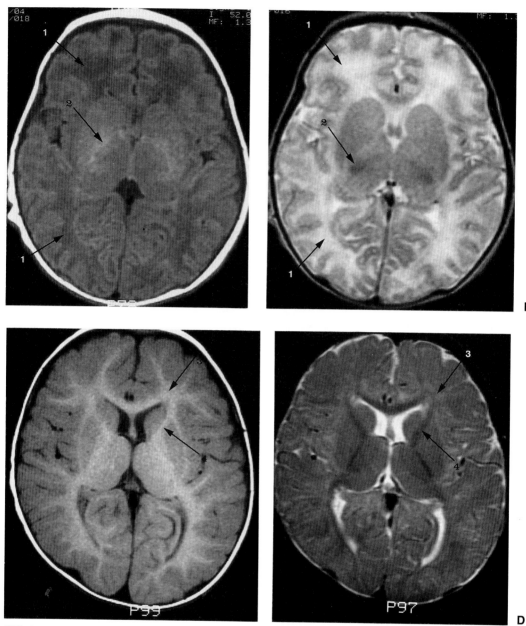

FIG. 21. Normal myelination for age. T1- (**A**) and T2-weighted (**B**) axial images of an 11-day-old term infant. Unmyelinated deep white matter tracts are hypointense on T1 and hyperintense on T2 weighting (*1*). Myelination of the posterior horns of the internal capsule is seen on both T1- and T2-weighted images (*2*, further progression on T1). T1- (**C**) and T2-weighted (**D**) axial images of a 12-month-old child. Myelination of the deep white matter tracks has progressed, appearing mature on T1, but remains immature on T2 weighting (*3*). Compare this with the mature adult brain (Fig. 1). The internal capsule, including the anterior limbs, now appears mature (*4*).

ously, the major determinant in formulating a differential diagnosis for an intracranial mass is the lesion's location. Thus, whether visualized by MRI or CT, the differential diagnosis is essentially the same. Some lesions have unique characteristics on MRI, however, that allow a shorter diagnostic list. Major intraaxial tumors are listed in Table 4. Extraaxial tumors appear in Table 5. A series of major differential diagnostic possibilities concerning tumors by their locations is presented in Tables 6 through 15. These lists are not meant to be exhaustive, but they offer a useful set of reasonable possibilities. Not considered here are other processes that can mimic a neoplastic process, including cerebritis, abscess, granuloma formation, demyelination, infarction, vascular abnormality, and hematoma. These possibilities also should be considered when the history and symptoms are suggestive. Each tumor will also be discussed separately in terms of its MRI characteristics, regardless of location.

Astrocytoma/Glioblastoma

This group consists of a histological spectrum of related intraaxial infiltrating tumors of glial origin. As a group, they are the most common intracranial neoplasms. The clinical prognosis worsens as the histological tumor grade increases from low- to high-grade astrocytoma with glioblastoma multiforme being the most malignant. Imaging characteristics also change with grade, but because of the large overlap of findings across tumor grades, MRI and CT are not reliable in grading a particular lesion. Biopsy is required.

Astrocytomas peak in the 20- to 50-year-old age group. They can occur anywhere in the brain but are usually supratentorial in adults and infratentorial in children. Involvement of the occipital lobes is unusual. When the brainstem is involved, the lesion is most often within the pons. The use of MRI demonstrates an intraaxial mass associated with variable edema. The mass typically is relatively homogeneous with a hyperintense signal on T2-weighted images. Little to no enhancement with gadolinium is seen with low-grade astrocytomas, and edema may be minimal. With higher grade astrocytomas, the degree of enhancement tends to increase, becoming nodular or ring-like (Fig. 26). Over time, a low-grade astrocytoma can become more aggressive, differentiating into a higher grade lesion. Calcification is present in a minority of cases, which is usually not seen on routine spin–echo sequences.

Glioblastoma multiforme is the most malignant of the glial tumors, and the prognosis is poor. It peaks later than astrocytomas, at about 50 years of age. Although it can occur anywhere in the brain, it favors the frontal and temporal lobes. It can cross the corpus callosum to involve the contralateral hemisphere, resulting in a butterfly appearance, termed butterfly glioma (Fig. 27). This appearance is not pathognomonic, however, because low-grade astrocytomas and lymphomas can also cross the corpus callosum.

Typically, MRI shows a heterogeneous mass with hemorrhage and necrosis. Marked edema extending along adjacent white matter tracts is

TABLE 5. *Major extraaxial masses*

Meningioma
Epidermoid
Dermoid
Lipoma
Arachnoid cyst
Metastasis
Lymphoma
Leukemia (to meninges)
Pituitary adenoma
Craniopharyngioma

TABLE 6. *Differential diagnosis of sellar neoplasms*

Pituitary adenoma
Craniopharyngioma
Meningioma
Chordoma
Metastasis
Aneurysm (mimicking a neoplasm)

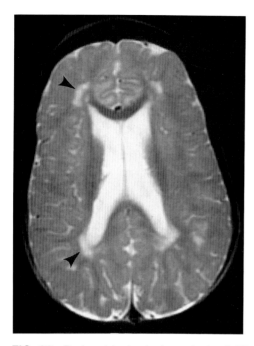

FIG. 22. Periventricular leukomalacia. A T2-weighted image demonstrates thinning of white matter tracts and persistent periventricular hyperintensity (*arrows*).

the rule. A glioblastoma is usually solitary. Thick nodular enhancement is seen on T1-weighted images after gadolinium administration. Gadolinium may also demonstrate abnormal enhancement along CSF pathways (ependyma and meninges) of the brain or spine, which is consistent with the spread of tumor. The major route for metastasis of a glioblastoma is CSF dissemination (drop mets). This can also occur with astrocytomas but is less common.

TABLE 7. *Differential diagnosis of suprasellar neoplasms*

Craniopharyngioma
Meningioma
Glioma (optic chiasm or hypothalamus)
Germ cell tumor
Epidermoid
Dermoid
Hamartoma of tuber cinereum
Arachnoid cyst
Aneurysm (mimicking a neoplasm)

TABLE 8. *Differential diagnosis of parasellar neoplasms*

Meningioma
Neurinoma (from cavernous sinus)
Metastasis
Epidermoid
Aneurysm (mimicking a neoplasm)

TABLE 9. *Differential diagnosis of pineal region neoplasm*

Pineocytoma
Pineoblastoma (PNET)
Germ cell tumors
Metastasis
Pineal cyst

TABLE 10. *Differential diagnosis of intraventricular neoplasms*

Ependymoma
Choroid plexus papilloma
Meningioma
Metastasis
Colloid cyst

TABLE 11. *Differential diagnosis of corpus callosum neoplasms*

Glioma
Lymphoma
Metastasis

TABLE 12. *Differential diagnosis of adult intraaxial posterior fossa neoplasms*

Metastasis
Hemangioblastoma (rare)

TABLE 13. *Differential diagnosis of childhood intraaxial posterior fossa neoplasms*

Cerebellar astrocytoma
Medulloblastoma (PNET)
Ependymoma
Brainstem glioma

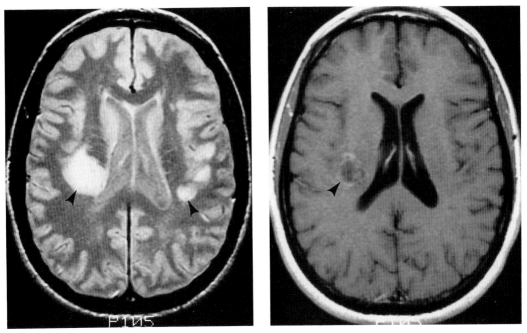

A   B

FIG. 23. Multiple sclerosis. **A:** A T2-weighted axial image demonstrates multiple hyperintense plaques of demyelination bilaterally (*arrows*). **B:** A T1-weighted axial image with gadolinium shows enhancement of the large plaque in the right periventricular white matter (*arrow*). This indicates active demyelination. The nonenhancing plaques on the left are old lesions not currently undergoing active demyelination.

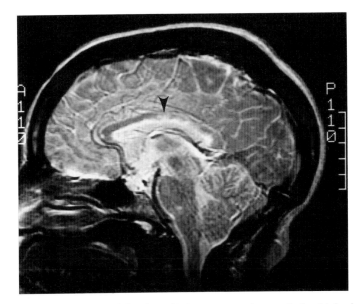

FIG. 24. Multiple sclerosis. A T2-weighted sagittal sequence demonstrates high-signal-intensity lesions extending into the corpus callosum. This is common in multiple sclerosis and rare in ischemic disease.

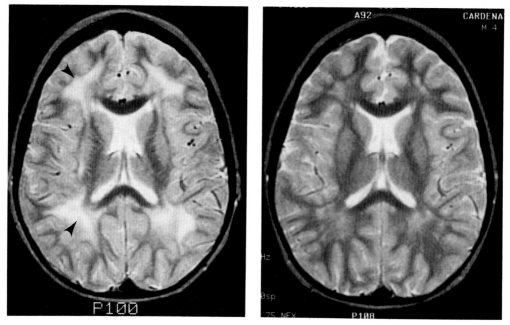

FIG. 25. Transient chemotherapy-induced leukoencephalopathy. **A:** A T2-weighted axial image shows diffuse hyperintensity throughout the deep white matter tracts *(arrows)* in a 4-year-old child receiving combination chemotherapy for acute lymphocytic leukemia. **B:** A T2-weighted axial image from a follow-up scan 1 month later shows marked improvement (decreased white matter signal).

Giant Cell Astrocytoma

A giant cell astrocytoma is a low-grade lesion associated with tuberous sclerosis. In this disorder, multiple nonenhancing cortical and subependymal tubers (hamartomas) are present that are isointense with the white matter. Occasionally, a subependymal tuber (usually near the foramen of Monro) will degenerate into a giant cell astrocytoma. These lesions enlarge and enhance with gadolinium (Fig. 28).

If the foramen of Monro is obstructed by a resulting mass effect, hydrocephalus develops.

Juvenile Pilocystic Astrocytoma (JPA)

A JPA is a relatively benign form of astrocytoma that occurs primarily in children. It does not have the infiltrating characteristics of the more aggressive astrocytomas, and if in a surgically accessible site, resection is curative. When supratentorial, JPAs are usually found

TABLE 14. *Differential diagnosis of cerebellopontine angle neoplasms*

Acoustic neurinoma
Meningioma
Epidermoid
Trigeminal neurinoma
Arachnoid cyst

TABLE 15. *Differential diagnosis of primary tumors with subarachnoid spread (drop mets)*

Medulloblastoma (PNET)
Ependymoma
Astrocytoma/glioblastoma
Germ cell tumors

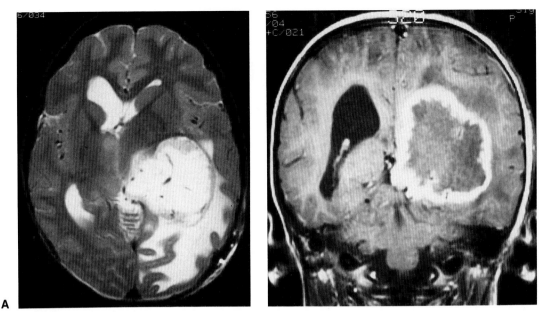

A

B

FIG. 26. Anaplastic astrocytoma. **A:** A T2-weighted axial image shows a large mass with some internal heterogeneity and a large amount of associated white matter edema (vasogenic edema). A mass effect causes subfalcine herniation and partial ventricular effacement. **B:** A coronal T1-weighted image with gadolinium shows relatively thick, nodular enhancement.

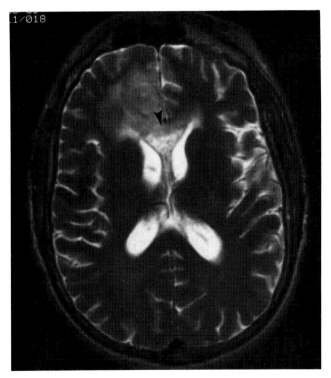

FIG. 27. Butterfly glioma. A T2-weighted image demonstrates a hyperintense lesion centered in the right frontal lobe but crossing the genu of the corpus callosum (*arrow*) to involve the left frontal lobe. The histologic finding was glioblastoma multiforme.

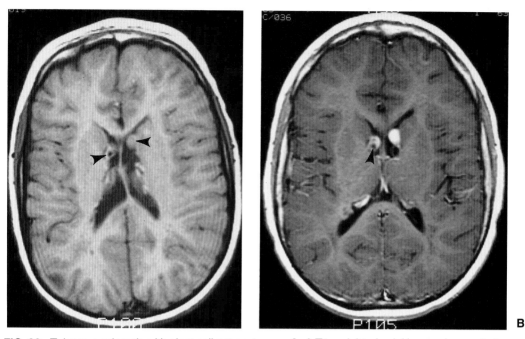

FIG. 28. Tuberous sclerosis with giant cell astrocytomas. **A:** A T1-weighted axial image demonstrates subependymal tubers (*arrows*). **B:** A T1-weighted image with gadolinium shows enhancement of both lesions and is consistent with degeneration to giant cell astrocytomas. The hypointense foci within the lesion on the right (*arrow*) were shown to be calcification on CT.

in the hypothalamus or optic system at or near the optic chiasm. These optic system gliomas are often associated with neurofibromatosis type I (the peripheral type, Fig. 29). Except for hypothalamic or chiasmatic lesions, a JPA typically contains a large cyst, often with an enhancing mural nodule (Fig. 30). In general, the lesion is hyperintense to adjacent brain on T2-weighted sequences, with little to no edema.

When infratentorial in location, JPAs most often involve the cerebellum, either the vermis or hemispheres. Approximately 80% of cerebellar astrocytomas in children are JPAs. The other 20% are the infiltrative type of astrocytoma. These ratios are reversed in the brainstem. Cerebellar lesions tend to displace the fourth ventricle and can cause hydrocephalus.

Oligodendroglioma

Another low-grade astrocytoma-like tumor that occurs mainly in adults is an oligodendroglioma. This intraaxial lesion tends to be superficial, favors the frontal lobes, is large at the time of diagnosis, and contains dense calcifications on CT. On MRI, the presence of calcification (and intratumor iron deposition) may cause the mass to have a low signal intensity on T2-weighted images. These lesions are usually hemorrhagic.

Ependymoma

When intracranial, ependymomas primarily occur in children and are infratentorial. They usually arise from the floor of the fourth ventricle, commonly extending into the foramina of Luschka and Magendie. They frequently result in obstructive hydrocephalus. When foraminal extension is present, this is highly suggestive that the mass is an ependymoma. Rarely, the tumor can arise supratentorially within the lateral ventricles or within the brain parenchyma (arising from ependymal cell rests).

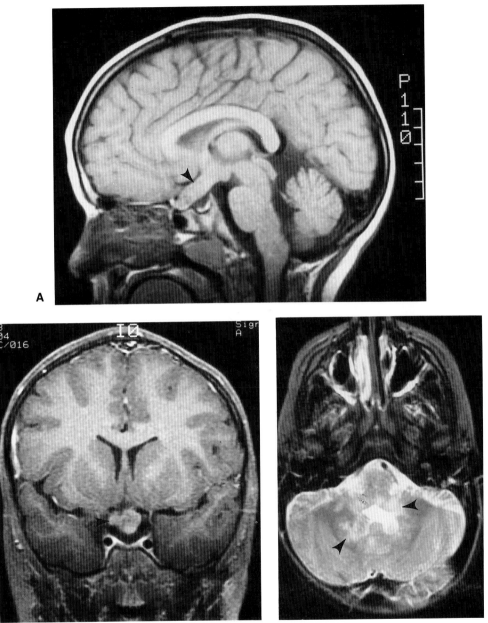

FIG. 29. Neurofibromatosis type I with optic chiasm glioma. **A:** A T1-weighted sagittal image demonstrates an optic chiasm (suprasellar) mass (*arrow*). **B:** A coronal T1-weighted image with gadolinium shows no enhancement of the mass, which also extends into the right optic nerve (*arrow*). **C:** A T2-weighted axial image through the posterior fossa demonstrates multiple hyperintense lesions in the cerebellar white matter and the middle cerebellar peduncles (*arrows*). These lesions represent hamartomatous changes, which are common in neurofibromatosis.

On MRI, ependymomas are heterogeneously hyperintense on T2-weighted sequences. They often contain cystic components, hemorrhage (bright on T1), and calcification. The latter is better seen with CT or by using a GRE MRI sequence. These tumors typically enhance, although in a heterogeneous pattern (Fig. 31). The heterogeneity can help in differentiating an ependymoma from a medulloblastoma because the latter tends to enhance homogeneously. Gadolinium enhancement is also useful in detecting subarachnoid spread of the tumor. Drop mets, which occur with ependymomas, are aggressive lesions of variable prognosis.

A subependymoma, in contrast, is an enhancing benign, well-marginated, solid mass that arises just beneath the ependymal lining, containing both ependymal and astrocytic elements. This lesion may be indistinguishable from an ependymoma on imaging studies, but it is rare, seldom calcifies, and occurs primarily during middle age.

Primitive Neuroectodermal Tumor (PNET)

The term PNET is given to a group of related tumors of undifferentiated neuroectodermal tissue. The major example in the posterior fossa is the medulloblastoma. Although rare, a cerebral neuroblastoma is the major supratentorial example. Both are aggressive lesions with a propensity for subarachnoid spread and drop mets. The supratentorial lesion occurs in young children and tends to have heterogeneous signal (Fig. 32) and enhancement with gadolinium. Typically, these are deep within the frontal or parietal lobes.

A medulloblastoma is a relatively common tumor with bimodal distribution, peaking around 5 and 20 years of age. It typically is positioned midline within the cerebellar vermis but may be paramedian within a cerebellar hemisphere. The mass commonly extends into the fourth ventricle, resulting in hydrocephalus. On CT, the lesion is characteristically high density and densely enhancing. Because of de-creased posterior fossa artifact and improved sensitivity in detecting subarachnoid spread (which is common), MRI is the diagnostic modality of choice.

On MRI, medulloblastomas typically are slightly hypointense to surrounding brain on T1 and mildly hyperintense on T2. They are often relatively homogeneous, but some heterogeneity with hemorrhage or cystic changes may be present. Calcification is rare, which may be useful in differentiating them from ependymomas. Intense enhancement with gadolinium is typical (Fig. 33). This lesion is highly malignant and, in addition to a subarachnoid spread of the tumor, may metastasize outside the CNS (e.g., to bone).

Hemangioblastoma

Hemangioblastomas are benign intraaxial tumors typically found in the cerebellum, but they also may occur in the medulla and spinal cord. They are generally solitary and occur in middle-aged adults, but when they are associated with von Hippel-Lindau syndrome, they may be multiple and occur at a younger age. Two-thirds of hemangioblastomas contain a cyst of varying signal intensities (isointense or hyperintense to the CSF on T1- and T2-weighted images). Characteristically, an enhancing nodule is present, superficially, abutting the pia (Fig. 34). Resection is curative if complete.

Metastasis

For the detection of CNS metastases, MRI has a greater sensitivity than does CT. Intraaxial metastases typically are hypointense or isointense with the surrounding brain on T1-weighted images, hyperintense on T2-weighted images, and enhance with gadolinium. Some are hemorrhagic (Table 1). They are often located at the gray–white junctions (regions of arteriolar narrowing). Massive surrounding edema, which follows deep white matter tracts (vasogenic edema), is the rule (Fig. 35). When multiple lesions are present, metastases are much more likely than is a primary tumor.

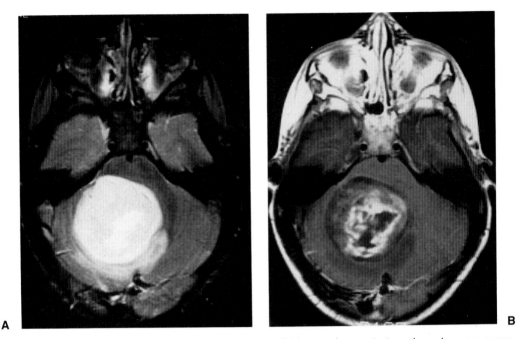

FIG. 30. Cerebellar astrocytoma. **A:** A T2-weighted axial image demonstrates a large homogeneous mass in the cerebellar vermis. The pons is compressed, and the fourth ventricle is effaced (obstructive hydrocephalus was present supratentorially). **B:** A T1-weighted image with gadolinium shows thick heterogeneous enhancement with central necrosis. No large cystic component was seen. This appearance suggests an infiltrating lesion, but the histologic finding was pilocystic astrocytoma.

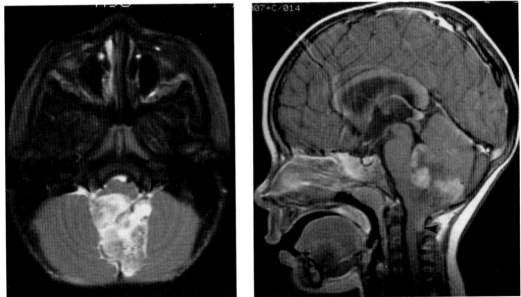

FIG. 31. Ependymoma. **A:** A T2-weighted axial image shows a heterogeneous, hyperintense midline mass in the posterior fossa (actually arising from the fourth ventricle). It compresses the midbrain and extends into the foramina of Luschka (*arrows*). **B:** A T1-weighted sagittal image with gadolinium shows the mass enhancing heterogeneously. Enhancing tumor is also seen filling the foramen of Magendie (*arrow*).

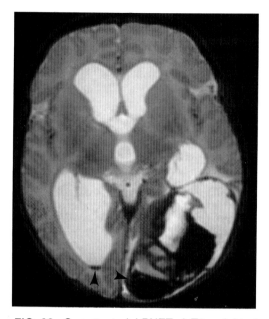

FIG. 32. Supratentorial PNET. A T2-weighted axial image demonstrates a large, heterogeneous parietooccipital tumor. The low-signal-intensity material within the lesion and the atrium of the right lateral ventricle (*arrows*) represents recent hemorrhage (intracellular methemoglobin). Hydrocephalus is present.

Extraaxial metastasis may involve the overlying bony calvarium (Fig. 36) or the meninges (causing intense enhancement, often indistinguishable from inflammatory meningitis, Fig. 15.) Bone metastases are best seen on T1-weighted images as the replacement of the normal bright fatty marrow with the relatively dark fluid-containing tumor. Primary tumors of bone, such as a clivus chordoma, have similar signal characteristics and can cause compression effects on the adjacent brain from bony expansion (Fig. 37).

Lymphoma

Primary CNS lymphoma (almost always non-Hodgkin's) is seen primarily in patients with AIDS. It usually presents as an intraaxial space-occupying mass. Most often, it is supratentorial, involving the basal ganglia, periventricular white matter, or corpus callosum. The lesions are multiple in approximately one half of patients and may be indistinguishable from metastases. They are rarely hemorrhagic and do not calcify. Edema is commonly present but, generally, is not as prominent a feature as with other primary neoplasms or metastases.

The signal characteristics of primary lymphoma are variable, ranging from isointense with the surrounding brain on both T1- and T2-weighted images to hyperintense on T2. The lesions often enhance homogeneously, although when associated with AIDS, ring enhancement is not unusual, making a differentiation from the lesions of toxoplasmosis difficult (Fig. 38). Usually, the CNS spread from systemic lymphoma is extraaxial, involving the meninges.

Choroid Plexus Papilloma

A choroid plexus papilloma is an uncommon intraventricular tumor that has a lobulated contour and, typically, is isointense to gray matter on T1 weighting and heterogeneously bright on T2. The lesion enhances with gadolinium and may contain calcification (dark on T2) and blood products from hemorrhage (Fig. 39). The tumor arises from the choroid plexus and is typically in a lateral ventricle in adults and in the fourth ventricle in children. A mass effect may expand the ventricle and block CSF outflow, causing hydrocephalus. Overproduction of CSF by the abnormal choroid plexus may also cause generalized hydrocephalus.

Colloid Cyst

This rare intraventricular lesion is diagnosed primarily by its characteristic location in the anterior roof of the third ventricle (Fig. 40). Its mucoid contents vary in constituents, resulting in variable signal characteristics, ranging from hypo- to hyperintense on T1- and T2-weighted images. It is nonenhancing. A colloid cyst is benign but may obstruct an adjacent foramen of Monro, causing hydrocephalus.

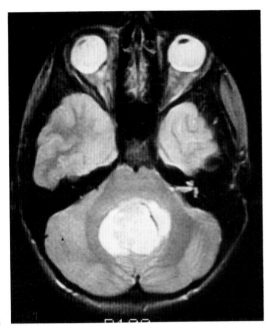

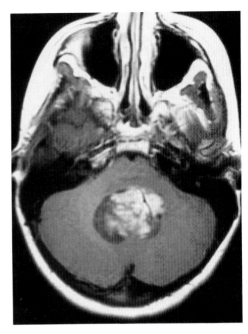

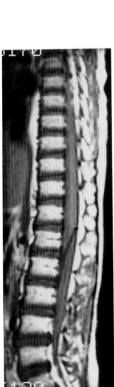

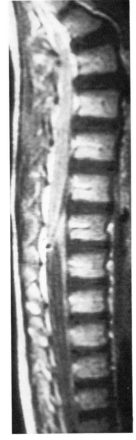

FIG. 33. Medulloblastoma. **A:** A T2-weighted axial image demonstrates a near-homogeneous vermian mass that distorts the pons and splays the middle cerebellar peduncles. **B:** A T1-weighted image with gadolinium shows intense, heterogeneous enhancement. T1-weighted midline thoracolumbar spine before (**C**) and after (**D**) administration of gadolinium shows intense enhancement along the spinal cord and throughout the thecal sac in the lumbosacral region. This represents extensive CSF spread of tumor (drop

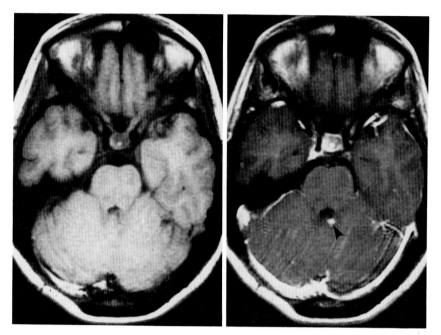

FIG. 34. Hemangioblastoma. T1-weighted axial images before and after gadolinium administration demonstrates a small enhancing vermian nodule (*arrow*). The patient had von Hippel-Lindau syndrome. (Courtesy of Todd Lempert, MD, Magnetic Imaging Affiliates).

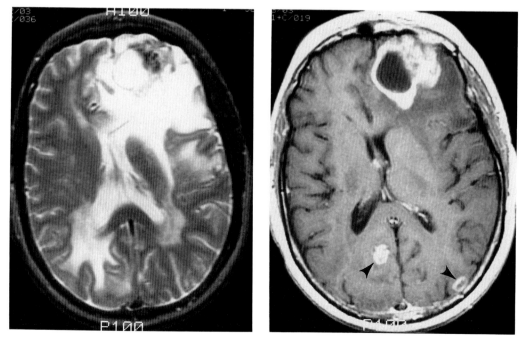

A   B

FIG. 35. Intraaxial metastasis (breast cancer). **A:** A T2-weighted axial image demonstrates a large left frontal mass with surrounding vasogenic edema. Edema is also present in the peritrigonal region on the right. **B:** A T1-weighted image with gadolinium demonstrates two additional masses posteriorly (*arrows*). All lesions are positioned at the gray–white junction.

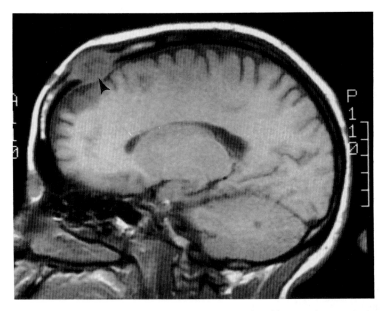

FIG. 36. Extraaxial metastasis (sarcoma). A sagittal T1-weighted image demonstrates an expansile mass in the frontal bone replacing the normal bright fatty marrow with an intermediate-signal-intensity tumor. A mass effect causes mild distortion of the underlying leptomeninges and brain (*arrow*).

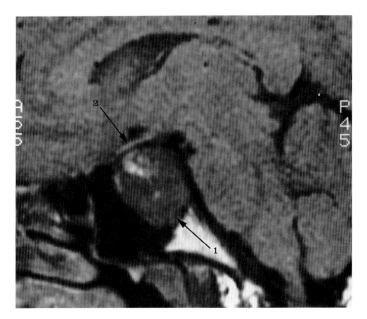

FIG. 37. Chordoma. A T1-weighted sagittal image demonstrates a large intermediate signal mass arising from the clivus (*1*), destroying the sella turcica. It impinges on the pituitary gland and elevates the optic chiasm (*2*).

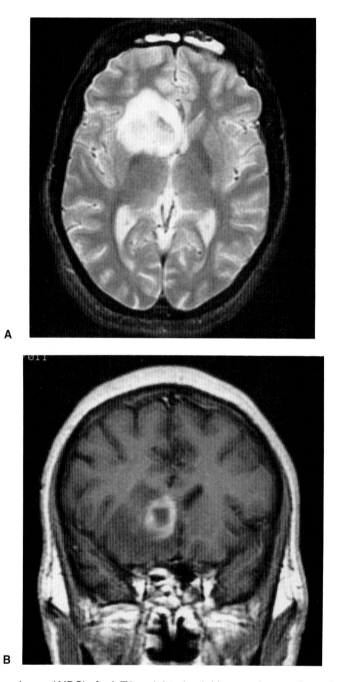

FIG. 38. CNS lymphoma (AIDS). **A:** A T2-weighted axial image shows a hyperintense mass with edema in the caudate nucleus on the right. **B:** A T1-weighted coronal image with gadolinium shows ring enhancement. This appearance is indistinguishable from that of toxoplasmosis (Fig. 17).

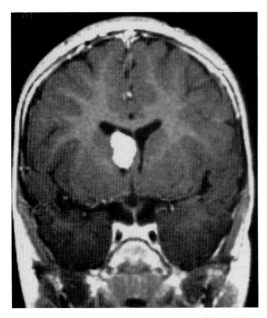

FIG. 39. Choroid plexus papilloma. A T1-weighted coronal image demonstrates an intensely enhancing, lobular mass arising from the choroid plexus on the right, near the foramen of Monro. No hydrocephalus is present.

Pineal Region Tumors

Tumors of the pineal gland are rare. Most are germ cell tumors with germinoma being the most frequent. This lesion typically occurs in adolescent boys and has a propensity for subarachnoid spread with drop mets. Pineal germinomas are well circumscribed, homogeneous lesions. Unless hemorrhage is present, they are often isointense with the adjacent brain on T1- and T2-weighted images and are best seen on sagittal sequences (Fig. 41). Intense homogeneous enhancement is expected. Heterogeneity with calcification (best seen on GRE) suggests a lesion other than a germinoma, such as a teratoma (Fig. 42). Intratumor fat is often seen in teratomas. These lesions should be differentiated from a pineal cyst, which is usually an asymptomatic, incidental finding. These are well-circumscribed, round lesions, which are bright on T2 (may not be isointense with CSF) and nonenhancing with gadolinium (Fig. 43).

Meningioma

The most common extraaxial, primary intracranial tumors are meningiomas. They typically have a broad dural base, often forming obtuse angles with the dura, and cause extrinsic compression on the adjacent brain. Common locations include parasagittal at the convexity, sphenoid wings, cerebellopontine angles, parasellar region, clivus, tentorium, and along the optic nerve sheaths (see Chapter 1, Fig. 6). Meningiomas rarely are intraventricular. The multiplanar capabilities of MRI are useful in demonstrating the extraaxial location of these lesions, which is of primary importance in formulating a differential diagnosis.

Meningiomas are commonly isointense to adjacent gray matter on both T1- and T2-weighted images, although this is variable, with some lesions being hyperintense on T2. Heterogeneity also varies with the degree of contained calcification (low signal) present, which is common. Virtually all meningiomas show intense, homogeneous enhancement with gadolinium (Fig. 44). These tumors commonly are circumscribed with visible vessels (vascular rim) along their interface with the adjacent brain. Edema occurs in approximately 50% of cases. They are usually benign and solitary and found in middle-aged and elderly adults. Multiple meningiomas are seen in association with neurofibromatosis type II (the central form).

Neurinoma

Two intracranial neurinomas that may be encountered are a trigeminal neurinoma and an acoustic neurinoma. The latter is more common, arising from the eighth cranial nerve, centered at the porus acusticus. Most of these tumors have an intracanalicular component that widens the internal auditory canal and a mass component extending into the cerebellopontine angle. This often compresses the adjacent pons or cerebellar hemisphere. These lesions are generally best imaged in the axial projection. Typically, a neurinoma is isointense with adjacent brain on T1-weighted images and hy-

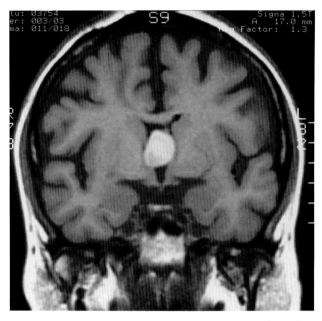

FIG. 40. Colloid cyst. A T1-weighted coronal image demonstrates a hyperintense, smoothly marginated mass arising from the anterior roof of the third ventricle.

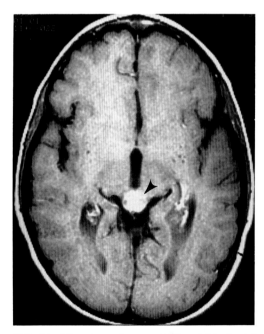

FIG. 41. Pineal germinoma. A T1-weighted axial image with gadolinium demonstrates a well-circumscribed, homogeneous intensely enhancing pineal mass (*arrow*) in an 11-year-old boy.

perintense on T2-weighted images. Intense enhancement with gadolinium is the rule (Fig. 45). The tumor may have cystic or hemorrhagic components. If present, these features, in addition to being centered at the porus acusticus, help differentiate an acoustic neurinoma from a meningioma, the major differential diagnostic consideration.

Bilateral acoustic neurinomas are associated with neurofibromatosis type II. Trigeminal neurinomas have imaging characteristics similar to those of acoustic neurinomas, except that they are positioned more anteriorly in the cerebellopontine angle and extend along the fifth cranial nerve into Meckel's cave (the posterior aspect of the cavernous sinus.)

Extraaxial Cysts

Arachnoid cysts, epidermoids, and dermoids are all benign lesions and are classified as cysts even though the latter two lesions are composed, at least in part, by the inclusion of solid material. These lesions are all nonvascular and show no enhancement with gadolinium.

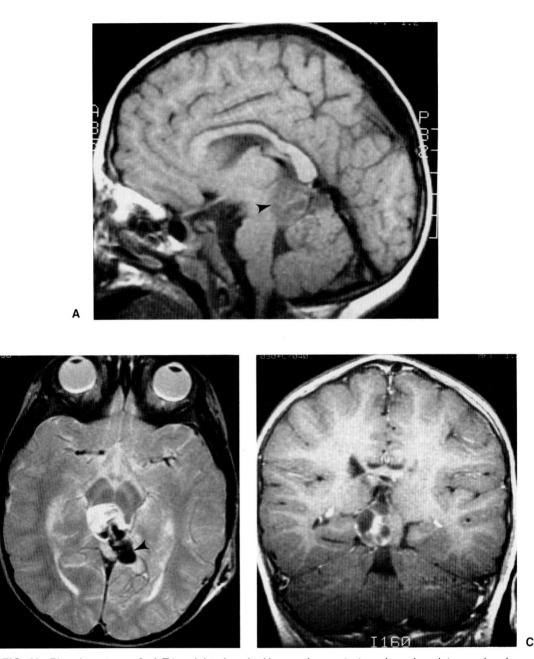

FIG. 42. Pineal teratoma. **A:** A T1-weighted sagittal image demonstrates a large hypointense pineal mass in a 6-year-old girl (*arrow*). **B:** T2-weighted axial images show a hyperintense lesion with a large low-signal-intensity component (*arrow*) shown by CT to represent calcification. **C:** A T1-weighted coronal image with gadolinium shows heterogeneity and partial enhancement. No fatty component is seen.

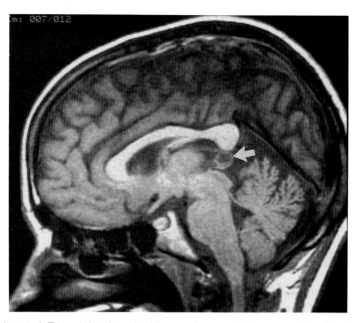

FIG. 43. Pineal cyst. A T1-weighted sagittal image demonstrates a small cyst in the pineal gland, which is isointense with the CSF (*arrow*).

An arachnoid cyst is a CSF-containing cyst within the arachnoid membrane that expands by CSF secretion, osmotic filtration, or a ball-valve mechanism. It may become symptomatic if sufficient compression of the adjacent brain results. Erosion and expansion of adjacent calvarium may occur. Arachnoid cysts are isointense with CSF on all standard imaging sequences (Fig. 46).

Epidermoid cysts contain slow-growing, ectopically located squamous epithelium. These are soft lobular lesions that typically conform to CSF spaces and adjacent brain. Preferred sites include the cerebellopontine angles, supra- or parasellar regions, and the middle cranial fossa. Typically, epidermoids are slightly hypointense to the CSF on T1-weighted images and slightly hyperintense on T2-weighted images (Fig. 47). Occasionally, they may be isointense to the CSF, making differentiation from an arachnoid cyst difficult.

Dermoid cysts are rare lesions resulting from embryonic cell rests. They contain multiple skin elements, including squamous epithelium, hair, fat, and sweat glands. Their fat content makes the diagnosis by MRI relatively specific, causing hyperintensity on T1 and relative signal loss on T2-weighted sequences (Fig. 48). The presence of fat can also be confirmed by signal loss on a fat saturation sequence. These lesions typically are seen in the parasellar region, within cisterns supratentorially or midline in the posterior fossa. If rupture occurs, fat globules (high signal intensity on T1) can be seen in the subarachnoid spaces, or intraventricular fat–fluid levels may occur.

Lipomas

Lipomas are benign fatty tumors that can be found within the subarachnoid spaces, which result from failure to reabsorb primitive meningeal tissue during embryogenesis. Although they may occur anywhere along the subarachnoid spaces, the pericallosal cistern is a favored location (Fig. 49) and is frequently associated with callosal dysgenesis. Lipomas are hyperintense on T1-weighted images and lose relative signal intensity on T2-weighted images. Signal loss during a fat saturation sequence is confirmatory. These lesions are typically asymptomatic.

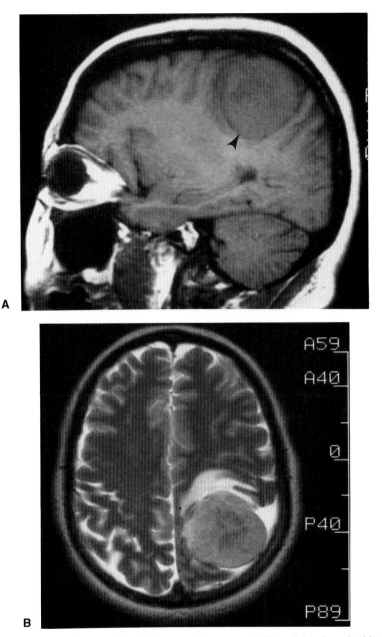

FIG. 44. Meningioma. **A:** A tumor in a 50-year-old woman. A T1-weighted sagittal image shows a large convexity mass, which is nearly isointense with adjacent gray matter (*arrow*). **B:** Same patient, a T2-weighted axial image shows the mass to be mildly hyperintense to the surrounding brain. Hyperintense edema extends into the adjacent white matter.

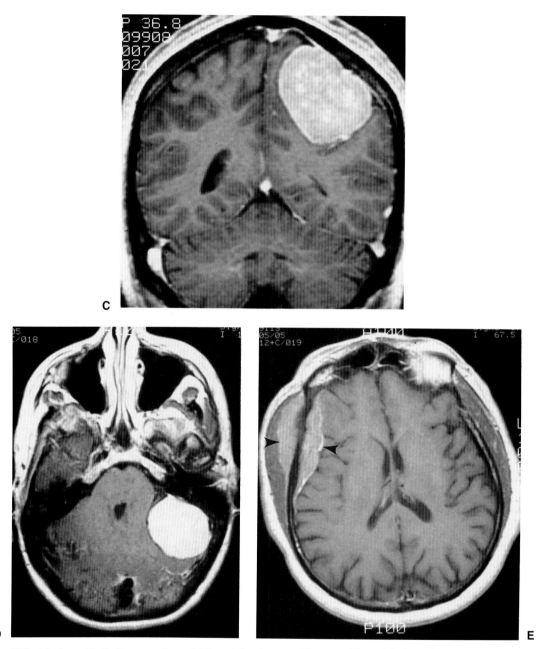

FIG. 44. *(contd.)* **C:** Same patient. A T1-weighted coronal image with gadolinium shows intense enhancement. This plane also demonstrates the tumor's broad dural base, indicating an extraaxial lesion. **D:** A T1-weighted axial image with gadolinium shows a homogeneously enhancing cerebellopontine angle meningioma in a 37-year-old woman. **E:** A T1-weighted axial image with gadolinium demonstrates a homogeneously enhancing *en plaque* meningioma in a 64-year-old man. The tumor has eroded through the calvarium, extending into the scalp *(arrows)*.

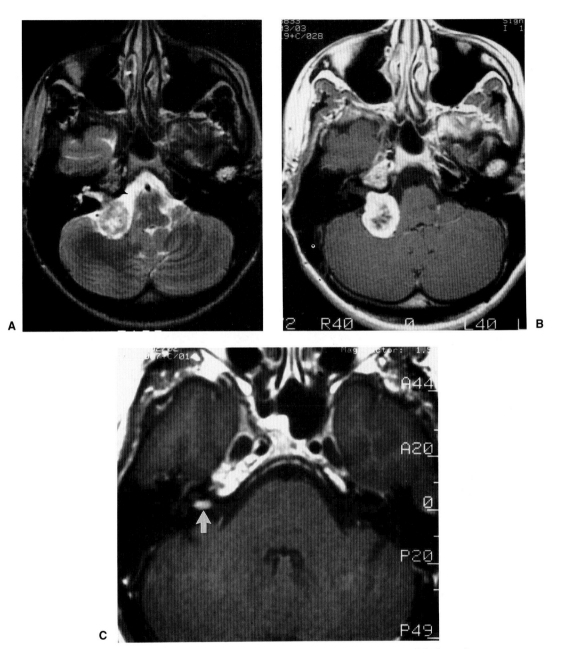

FIG. 45. Acoustic neurinoma. **A:** A T2-weighted axial image demonstrates a mildly hyperintense mass at the cerebellopontine angle in a 32-year-old woman. The tumor extends along the seventh/eighth nerve complex into the porus acusticus (*arrow*). **B:** A T1-weighted image with gadolinium shows intense enhancement and a central nonenhancing region of fluid or necrosis. **C:** A T1-weighted axial image with gadolinium in another patient demonstrates a small, intensely enhancing intracanalicular acoustic neuroma (*arrow*).

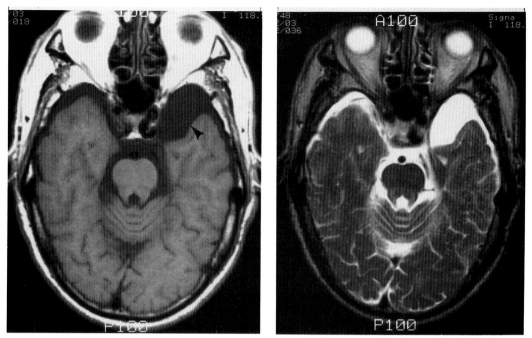

FIG. 46. Arachnoid cyst. **A:** A T1-weighted axial image demonstrates a homogeneous extraaxial cyst, isointense with the CSF, positioned anterior to the left temporal lobe (*arrow*). The mass effect alters the brain's contour. **B:** A T2-weighted image shows the cyst to remain isointense with the CSF.

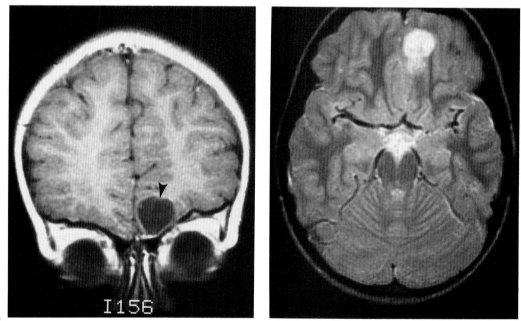

FIG. 47. Epidermoid. **A.** A T1-weighted coronal image demonstrates a homogeneous, extraaxial hypointense mass (*arrow*) along the left skull base. **B:** A T2-weighted axial image shows homogeneous hyperintensity, isointense with the CSF. When isointense to the CSF, these lesions are difficult to differentiate from arachnoid cysts.

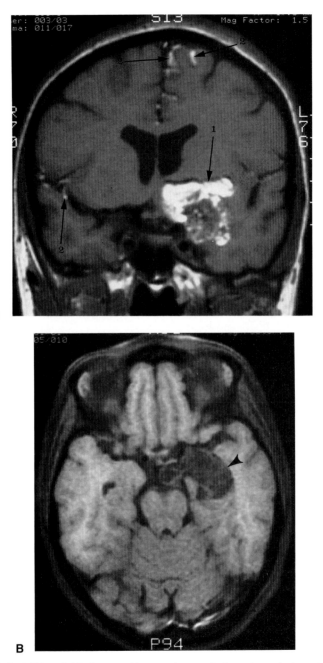

FIG. 48. Dermoid. **A:** A T1-weighted coronal image demonstrates a large heterogeneous, left parasellar mass (*1*). The high-signal-intensity material within the mass is fat. Lesion rupture has occurred in this case, resulting in high-signal-intensity fat globules within the CSF along multiple sulci (*2*). **B:** A T1-weighted fat saturation axial image shows disappearance of the lesion's high signal component (*arrow*). This confirms that the hyperintense material visualized was fat and not blood products.

Pituitary Adenoma

The pituitary gland is best evaluated with T1-weighted images in the coronal and sagittal projections. The normal anterior pituitary (adenohypophysis) is isointense with gray matter and can measure up to 1 cm craniocaudally. The infundibulum (stalk) can be seen extending cephalad to the hypothalamus. The posterior pituitary (neurohypophysis) appears as a "bright spot" in the posterior sella turcica (Fig. 50).

Pituitary adenomas are benign, slow-growing tumors of the anterior pituitary gland. Hormonally active lesions tend to present early, when the lesion is less than 10 mm, and classified by size as a microadenoma. Macroadenomas are lesions greater than 10 mm in size. They tend to be hormonally inactive and present later with symptoms of optic chiasm compression.

Microadenomas can be subtle. They are usually slightly hypointense with the normal gland on T1-weighted sequences and variable (often more subtle) on T2 weighting. Other clues to the presence of a microadenoma include a contour abnormality (coronal), such as an asymmetric bulge or convexity, and contralateral deviation of the infundibulum (Fig. 51). In difficult cases, gadolinium administration may be useful because the normal gland tends to enhance to a greater degree than the microadenoma, improving its conspicuousness.

Macroadenomas tend to be more heterogeneous because they contain hemorrhage (bright T1) and cystic degeneration (bright T2, Fig. 52). Important considerations with these lesions include an evaluation for invasion of the cavernous sinus, erosion of the sphenoid sinus, and suprasellar extension with impingement on the optic chiasm.

Craniopharyngioma

Craniopharyngiomas are benign lesions consisting of Rathke's cleft cell remnants. They are suprasellar in location and vary in size from tiny to several centimeters. There is a bimodal age distribution with the lesions occurring in childhood and middle age. Patients present with headache or visual disturbances. Typically, there is a solid and a cystic component to the lesion. The solid portion is heterogeneous with an increased signal on T1-weighted images and enhances with gadolinium. The cystic component is homogeneous, hyperintense on T2, and is nonenhancing (Fig. 53).

A Rathke's cleft cyst can mimic a craniopharyngioma but tends to be small, intrasellar, isointense with the CSF on all sequences, and nonenhancing. These lesions are usually asymptomatic, incidental findings.

Postoperative Tumor Evaluation

Four to 6 weeks after an operative resection of an intracranial tumor, a baseline scan including a T1, T2, and gadolinium-enhanced T1-weighted sequences should be obtained. The use of gadolinium is an important step because, even if the original tumor was nonenhancing, the recurrent tumor usually is. When tumor is found, the recurrence is usually seen in the postoperative tumor bed. Signs of recurrence include increasing distortion or mass effect and new enhancement at the operative site (Fig. 54). Postoperatively, the meninges tend to enhance and appear thick but are smooth in the absence of recurrence. If involved with recurrent tumor, a lumpy meningeal contour is often seen, causing distortion of the adjacent brain.

DEVELOPMENTAL ABNORMALITIES

The development of the brain is a complex process that begins with the closure of the neural tube during the 4th week of gestation and extends beyond the neonatal period. Ischemic, metabolic, or infectious insults to the brain during embryogenesis can result in a number of malformations, which may be supra- or infratentorial and involve gray or white matter tracts.

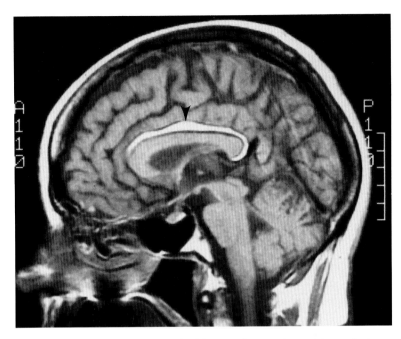

FIG. 49. Callosal lipoma. A T1-weighted sagittal image shows a hyperintense lesion conforming to the contour of the corpus callosum (*arrow*). No callosal dysgenesis is present in this case.

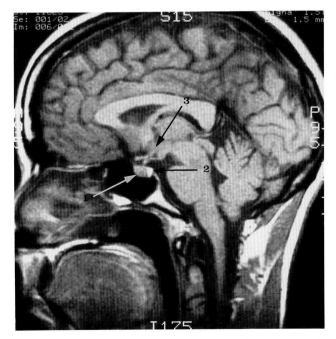

FIG. 50. Normal pituitary gland. A T1-weighted sagittal image demonstrates the adenohypophysis (*1*), which is isointense with the gray matter, and the hyperintense neurohypophysis (*2*). The infundibulum connects the pituitary gland to the hypothalamus (*3*).

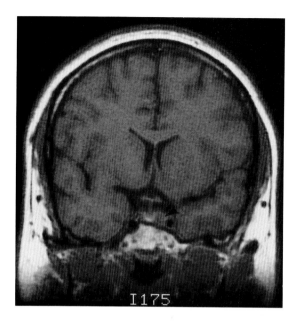

FIG. 51. Pituitary microadenoma. A T1-weighted coronal image demonstrates a small mass in the left aspect of the pituitary, which is hypointense to the rest of the gland (*arrow*). A mass effect is causing contralateral deviation of the infundibulum (stalk).

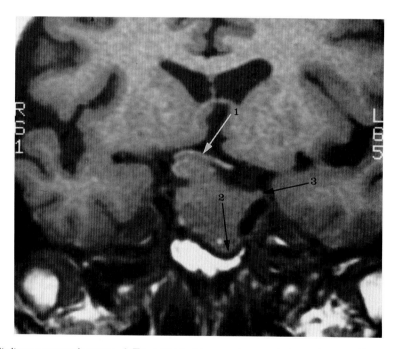

FIG. 52. Pituitary macroadenoma. A T1-weighted image demonstrates a large sellar mass that extends into the suprasellar region to distort the contour of the optic chiasm (*1*). The tumor depresses the sellar floor (*2*). Invasion of the cavernous sinus on the left (*3*) is also likely.

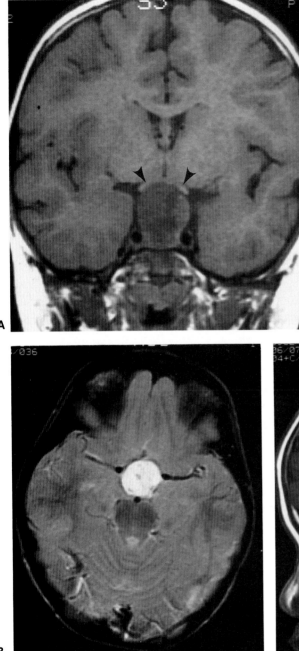

FIG. 53. Craniopharyngioma. **A:** A T1-weighted coronal image demonstrates a large, hypointense suprasellar mass. It extends inferiorly into the sella and, superiorly, to impinge on the optic chiasm, distorting its contour (*arrows*). The homogeneous hypointensity is somewhat unusual. **B:** A T2-weighted axial image shows a hyperintense cystic portion with a small amount of heterogeneous intermediate-signal-intensity material centrally, representing solid tissue. **C:** A T1-weighted sagittal image with gadolinium shows heterogeneous enhancement of the solid material within the lesion (*arrow*).

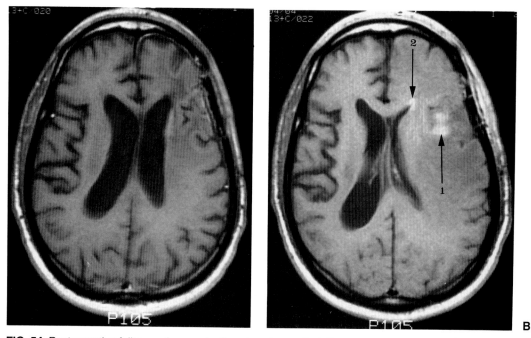

FIG. 54. Postoperative follow-up for anaplastic astrocytoma. **A:** A T1-weighted axial image with gadolinium 6 weeks after surgery shows mild distortion and low-signal-intensity encephalomalacia in the left frontoparietal region. This is consistent with previous surgery. No gadolinium enhancement is seen within the brain to suggest any residual or recurrent tumor. **B:** A T1-weighted image with gadolinium on subsequent follow-up shows a mass effect with sulcal effacement and intraparenchymal enhancement (*1*). This is consistent with tumor recurrence. The enhancing margin along the frontal horn of the left lateral ventricle (*2*) indicates subependymal spread of tumor.

Dysgenesis of the Corpus Callosum

Formation of the corpus callosum occurs during 8 to 20 weeks of gestational age. Evaluation of this structure is important because callosal dysgenesis is associated with a wide variety of other congenital brain anomalies, including gray matter migrational abnormalities and Dandy-Walker and Chiari malformations. The corpus callosum forms anteriorly from the genu, progressing posteriorly through the body to the splenium. The rostrum (anterior) forms last. Thus, when an insult occurs during formation, it always affects the posterior aspect of the callosum and the rostrum, resulting in, at least partial agenesis. If the insult occurs early enough in formation, complete agenesis of the corpus callosum may occur.

Because posterior absence is always a part in callosal dysgenesis, a relative deficiency in posterior periventricular white matter results, causing compensatory dilatation of the ventricular atria, called colpocephaly. The absence of callosal tissue also allows the third ventricle to be "high riding," extending between the lateral ventricles into the intrahemispheric fissure. This is called an intrahemispheric cyst. The sagittal plane is best for evaluating callosal formation (Fig. 55). Colpocephaly is best seen in the axial plane; the presence of an intrahemispheric cyst is best seen on coronal sections. The normal corpus callosum appears thin at birth but thickens after birth as myelination of its fibers occurs.

Neuronal Migration Anomalies

Beginning in the 8th week of gestation, the cortical gray matter is formed by migration from the germinal matrix (which is periventricular in location) to the cortical surface. By the 28th week, the brain loses its smooth, agyric appearance with developing sulcation, which

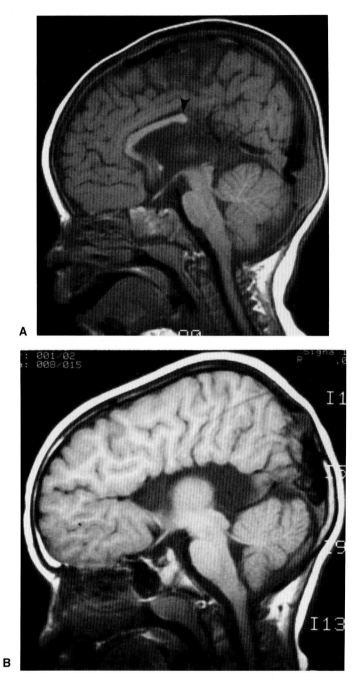

FIG. 55. Agenesis of the corpus callosum. **A:** A T1-weighted sagittal image demonstrates partial dysgenesis of the corpus callosum. The genu is intact, but development was arrested at the posterior body (*arrow*), resulting in the absence of the splenium. **B:** A T1-weighted sagittal image demonstrating complete agenesis of the corpus callosum.

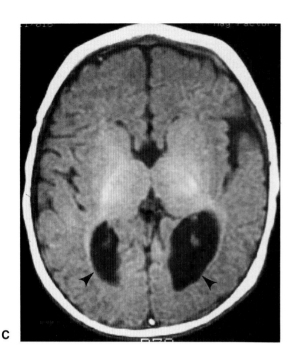

FIG. 55. *(contd.)* **C:** A T1-weighted axial image demonstrates colpocephaly (*arrows*), which is the dilatation of the ventricular atria seen in callosal agenesis because of a posterior deficiency of adjacent white matter tracts.

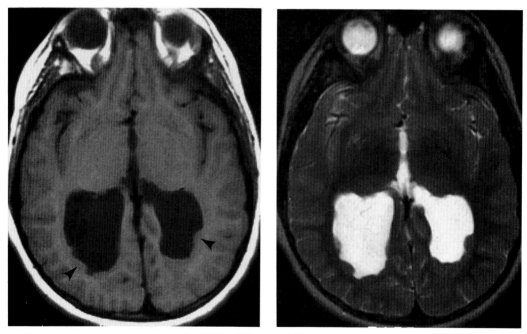

FIG. 56. Heterotopic gray matter. **A:** A T1-weighted axial image reveals a nodular appearance to the lining of the ventricular atria (*arrows*). These nodules are isointense with cortical gray matter and represent a migration arrest. **B:** A T2-weighted image demonstrates that the periventricular nodules remain isointense with cortical gray matter.

is completed and in an adult pattern at pregnancy term.

An insult to the germinal matrix during neuronal migration can cause a migrational arrest, resulting in heterotopic gray matter (normal gray matter in an abnormal location). Early arrest can result in focal nodular-like gray matter heterotropias. These are usually seen along the lateral ventricles, either subependymal or within the periventricular white matter. Because they represent foci of normal gray matter (albeit in an abnormal location), they will be isointense with gray matter on all sequences (Fig. 56). The major differential diagnostic consideration is tuberous sclerosis; however, in the latter condition, the subependymal hamartomas are typically isointense with white matter rather than gray matter. Patients with heterotopic gray matter usually present with seizures.

A more serious abnormality of neuronal migration results in agyria (lissencephaly) or pachygyria. In these conditions, the neuronal migration is arrested subcortically, involving a large area of brain. This results in undersulcation, giving the affected surface a smooth flat appearance (Fig. 57). In addition to seizures, these patients suffer from mental retardation.

Polymicrogyria is clinically less severe than agyria or pachygyria but has a similar, smooth appearance with few, flat gyri. If present, adjacent gliosis and anomalous draining veins can help differentiate this condition from pachygyria. In polymicrogyria, the migrating neurons reach the cortex but are arranged abnormally.

Schizencephaly is a condition in which gray matter-lined clefts extend from the lateral ventricles to the cortical surface. This should be differentiated from porencephaly, which is a result of focal brain destruction. Both have a communication with the lateral ventricles, but only schizencephaly has walls lined with gray matter (Fig. 58).

Posterior Fossa Anomalies

An insult to the developing cerebellum and fourth ventricle can result in cerebellar hypoplasia and a Dandy-Walker malformation or variant. The findings in a Dandy-Walker malformation include a superior attachment of the tentorium, resulting in a large posterior fossa. The vermis is absent (agenetic), enlarging the fourth ventricle which communicates with the cisterna magna (Fig. 59). Most patients also have hydrocephalus. A Dandy-Walker variant has vermian tissue present, albeit dysgenetic, and the posterior fossa may not be enlarged.

An Arnold-Chiari II malformation is associated with an inferior tentorial attachment and a small posterior fossa. The cerebellar tonsils, and often the vermis and medulla, herniate through the foramen magnum into the cervical canal, often causing a cervicomedullary kink. The cerebellar hemispheres appear to wrap around the brainstem (called the "banana sign" in obstetrical ultrasound images) and beaking of the tectum occurs (Fig. 60). The falx is often fenestrated and interdigitation of gyri occur. Most patients have concurrent hydrocephalus. Many also have callosal dysgenesis. Virtually all patients with a Chiari II malformation have a meningomyelocele.

A Chiari I malformation is a condition in which the cerebellar tonsils extend greater than 2 mm below the foramen magnum. The symptoms depend on the extent of tonsillar ectopia. The cervical cord should also be examined because approximately 20% of these patients will have a syrinx (Fig. 61).

Encephaloceles

Encephaloceles may be occipital, frontoethmoidal, and rarely, parietal or sphenoidal. This condition is not a result of brain maldevelopment, but rather, it is a calvarial defect that allows herniation of the brain and meninges extracranially (Fig. 62).

BIBLIOGRAPHY

Books

1. Atlas SW. *Magnetic resonance imaging of the brain and spine.* New York: Raven Press; 1991.
2. Barkovich AJ. *Pediatric neuroimaging.* New York: Raven Press; 1990.

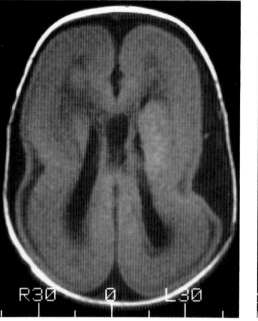

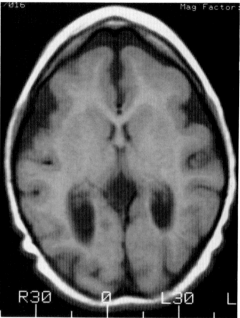

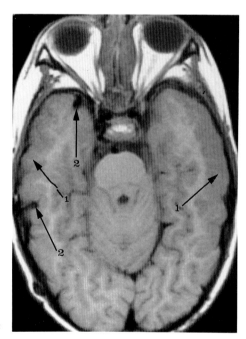

FIG. 57. Neuronal migration abnormalities. **A:** Agyria. A T1-weighted axial image demonstrates a smooth brain surface with total absence of gyri and sulci. **B:** Pachygyria. A T1-weighted image shows diminished sulcation. The gyri are broad and smooth with thickened cortical gray matter. **C:** Polymicrogyria. A T1-weighted axial image shows a smooth pachygyric-type cortex along the temporal lobes bilaterally (*1*). Anomalous draining veins (*2*) help differentiate polymicrogyria from pachygyria.

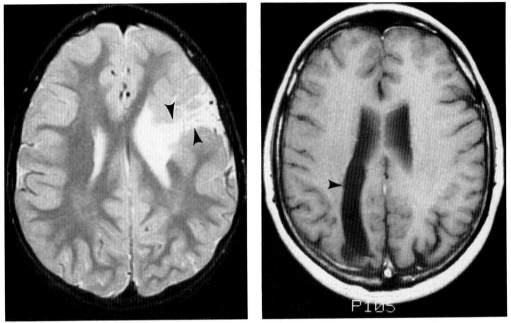

FIG. 58. A: Schizencephaly. A T2-weighted axial image demonstrates a gray matter-lined, CSF-containing cleft (*arrows*) extending from the left lateral ventricular body to the cortical surface. **B:** Porencephaly. A T1-weighted axial image demonstrates a CSF-containing cleft extending beyond the ventricular margins into the brain parenchyma (in this case, extension is to the cortical surface). Unlike schizencephaly, a porencephalic cyst or cleft extends into white matter without a gray matter lining (*arrow*).

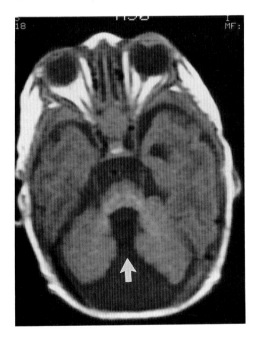

FIG. 59. Dandy-Walker malformation. A T1-weighted axial image demonstrates the absence of the cerebellar vermis and direct communication of the fourth ventricle with the cisterna magna (*arrow*). The cerebellar hemispheres appear characteristically splayed laterally.

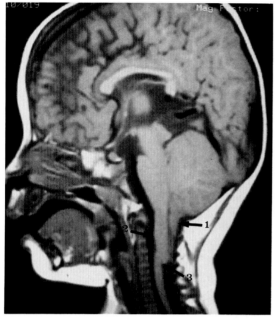

FIG. 60. Arnold-Chiari II malformation. **A:** A T1-weighted sagittal image demonstrates herniation of the cerebellar tonsils (*1*) and medulla (*2*) through the foramen magnum into the cervical canal, causing a cervicomedullary kink (*3*). **B:** A T1-weighted axial image shows complete effacement of the fourth ventricle. The cerebellum also appears to wrap around the brainstem (*arrows*). **C:** A T1-weighted axial image near the vertex shows fenestration of the falx with interdigitating gyri (*arrows*).

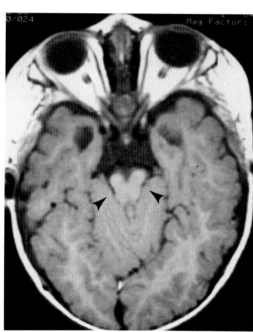

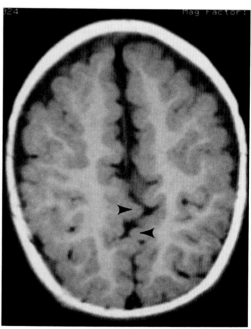

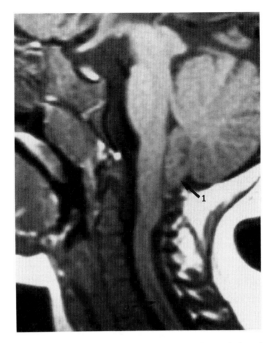

FIG. 61. Chiari I malformation. A T1-weighted sagittal image demonstrates extension of the cerebellar tonsils (*1*) through the foramen magnum (greater than 2 mm). A syrinx is also present in the cervical cord (*2*).

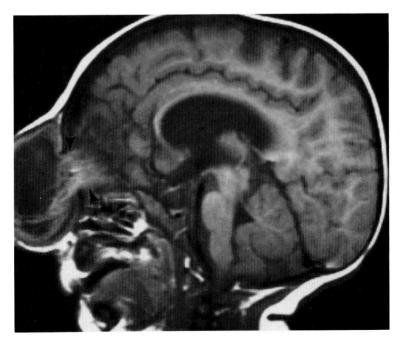

FIG. 62. Frontoethmoidal encephalocele. A T1-weighted sagittal image demonstrates a calvarial defect (*arrows*) through which brain and meninges extend extracranially.

Journals

1. Drayer BP. Imaging of the aging brain. Part I. Normal findings. *Radiology* 1988;166:785–796.

2. Drayer BP. Imaging of the aging brain. Part II. Pathological conditions. *Radiology* 1988;166:797–806.

3. Jungreis CA, Kanal E, Hirsch WL, Martinez AJ, Moosey J. Normal perivascular spaces mimicking lacunar infarction: MR imaging. *Radiology* 1988;169:101–104.

4. Sato A, Takahashi S, Soma Y, Ishii K, Kikuchi Y, Watanabe T, Sakamoto K. Cerebral infarction: early detection by means of contrast-enhanced cerebral arteries at MR imaging. *Radiology* 1991;178:433–439.

5. Hesselink JR, Dowd CF, Healy ME, Hajek P, Baker LL, Luerssen TG. MR imaging of brain contusions: a comparative study with CT. *AJR Am J Roentgenol* 1988;150:1133–1142.

6. Atlas SW, Mark AS, Grossman RI, Gomori JM. Intracranial hemorrhage; gradient-echo MR imaging at 1.5T. *Radiology* 1988;168:803–807.

7. Atlas SW, Mark AS, Fram EK, Grossman RI. Vascular intracranial lesions: applications of gradient-echo MR imaging. *Radiology* 1988;169:455–461.

8. Nadel L, Braun IF, Kraft KA, Fatouros PP, Laine FJ. Intracranial vascular abnormalities: value of MR phase imaging to distinguish thrombus from flowing blood. *AJNR Am J Neuroradiol* 1990;11:1133–1140.

9. Lemme-Plaghos L, Kucharczyk W, Brant-Zawadzki M, Uske A, Edwards M, Norman D, Newton TH. MRI of angiographically occult vascular malformations. *AJR Am J Roentgenol* 1986;146:1223–1228.

10. Sze G, Krol G, Olsen WL, Harper PS, Galicich JH, Heier LA, Zimmerman RD, Deck MD. Hemorrhagic neoplasms: MR mimics of occult vascular malformations. *AJR Am J Roentgenol* 1987;149:1223–1230.

11. Halmes AB, Zimmerman RD, Morgello S, Weingarten K, Becker RD, Jennis R, Deck MDF. MR imaging of brain abscesses. *AJR Am J Roentgenol* 1989;152:1073–1085.

12. Chang KH, Han MN, Roh JK, Kim IO, Han MC, Kim CW. Gd-DPTA-enhanced MR imaging of the brain in patients with meningitis: comparison with CT. *AJR Am J Roentgenol* 1990;154:809–816.

13. Tien RD, Chu PK, Hesselink JR, Duberg A, Wiley C. Intracranial cryptococcosis in immunocompromised patients: CT and MR findings in 29 cases. *AJR Am J Roentgenol* 1991;156:1245–1251.

14. Ramsey RG, Geremia GK. CNS complications of AIDS: CT and MRI findings. *AJR Am J Roentgenol* 1988;151:449–454.

15. Balakrishnan J, Becker PS, Kumar AJ, Zinreich SJ, McArthur JC, Bryan RN. Acquired immunodeficiency syndrome: correlation of radiologic and pathologic findings in the brain. *Radiographics* 1990;10:201–215.

16. Teitelbaum GP, Otto RJ, Lin M, Watanabe AL, Stull MA, Manz HJ, Bradley WG. MR imaging of neuro cysticercosis. *AJR Am J Roentgenol* 1989;153:857–866.

17. Barkovich AJ, Kjos BO, Jackson DE, Norman D. Normal maturation of the neonatal and infarct brain: MR imaging at 1.5 T. *Radiology* 1988;166:173–180.

18. Mark AS, Atlas SW. Progressive multifocal leukoencephalopathy in patients with AIDS: appearance on MR images. *Radiology* 1989;173:517–520.

19. Barkovich AJ, Truwit CL. Brain damage from perinatal asphyxia: correlation of MR findings with gestational age. *AJNR Am J Neuroradiol* 1990;11:1087–1096.

20. Flodmark O, Lupton B, Li D, et al. MR imaging of periventricular leukomalacia in childhood. *AJNR Am J Neuroradiol* 1989;10:111–118.

21. Nesbit GM, Forbes GS, Scheithauer BW, Okazaki H, Rodriguez M. Multiple sclerosis: histopathologic and MR and/or CT correlation in 37 cases at biopsy and three cases at autopsy. *Radiology* 1991;180:467–474.

22. Barkhof F, Scheltens P, Frequin STFM, Nauta JJP, Tas MW, Valk J, Hommes OR. Relapsing-remitting multiple sclerosis: sequential enhances MR imaging vs. clinical findings in determining disease activity. *AJR Am J Roentgenol* 1992;159:1041–1047.

23. Gean-Marton AD, Vezina LG, Marton KI, Stimac GK, Peyster RG, Taveras JM, Davis KR. Abnormal corpus callosum: a sensitive and specific indicator of multiple sclerosis. *Radiology* 1991;180:215–221.

24. Dooms GC, Hecht S, Brant-Zawadzki M, Berthiaume Y, Norman D, Newton TH. Brain radiation lesions: MR imaging. *Radiology* 1986;158:149–155.

25. Ebner F, Ranner G, Slavc I, Urban C, Kleinert R, Radner H, Einspieler R, Justich E. MR findings in methotrexate-induced CNS abnormalities. *AJNR Am J Neuroradiol* 1989;10:959–964.

26. Wilson DA, Ruprecht N, Bowman ME, Chaffin MJ, Sexauer CL, Prince JR. Transient white matter changes on MR images in children undergoing chemotherapy for acute lymphocytic leukemia: correlation with neuropsychologic deficiencies. *Radiology* 1991;180:205–209.

27. Dean BL, Drayer BP, Bird CR, Flom RA, Hodak JA, Coons SW, Carey RG. Gliomas: classification with MR imaging. *Radiology* 1990;174:411—415.

28. Altman NR, Purser RK, Post MJ. Tuberous sclerosis: characteristics at CT and MR imaging. *Radiology* 1988;167:527–532.

29. Lee Y, Van Tassel P, Bruner JM, Moser RP, Share JC. Juvenile pilocytic astrocytomas: CT and MRI characteristics. *AJR Am J Roentgenol* 1989;152:1263–1270.

30. Aoki S, Barkovich AJ, Nishimura K, Kjos BO, Machida T, Cogen P, Edwards M, Norman D. Neurofibromatosis types 1 and 2: cranial MR findings. *Radiology* 1989;172:527–534.

31. Lee Y, Van Tassel P. Intracranial oligodendrogliomas: imaging findings in 35 untreated cases. *AJNR Am J Neuroradiol* 1989;10:119–127.

32. Spoto GP, Press GA, Hesselink JR, Solomon M. Intracranial ependymoma and subependymoma: MR manifestations. *AJR Am J Neuroradiol* 1990;154:837–845.

33. Figeroa RE, el Gammal T, Brooks BS, Holgate R, Miller W. MR findings on primitive neuro ectodermal tumors. *J Comput Assist Tomogr* 1989;13:773–778.

34. Buetow PC, Smirniotopoulos JG, Dane S. Congenital brain tumors: a review of 45 cases. *AJR Am J Roentgenol* 1990;155:587–593.

35. Lee SR, Sanches J, Mark AS, Dillon WP, Norman D, Newton TH. Posterior fossa hemangioblastomas: MR imaging. *Radiology* 1989;171:463–468.

36. Claussen C, Laniado M, Schorner W, Niendorf HP, Weinmann HJ, Fiegler W, Felix R. Gadolinium-DTPA in MR imaging of glioblastomas and intracranial metastases. *AJNR Am J Neuroradiol* 1985;6:669–674.

37. Schwaighofer BW, Hesselink JR, Press GA, Wolf RL, Healy ME, Berthothy DP. Primary intracranial CNS lymphoma: MR manifestations. *AJNR Am J Neuroradiol* 1989;10:725–729.

38. Coates TL, Hinshaw DB Jr, Peckman N, Thompson JR, Hasso AN, Holshouser BA, Knierim DS. Pediatrics choroid plexus neoplasms: MR, CT and pathologic correlation. *Radiology* 1989;173:81–88.

39. Maeder PP, Holtas SL, Basibuyuk LN, Salford LG, Tapper UA, Brun A. Colloid cysts of the third ventricle: correlation of MR and CT findings with histology and chemical analysis. *AJR Am J Roentgenol* 1990; 155:135–141.

40. Tien RD, Barkovich AJ, Edwards MS. MR imaging of pineal tumors. *AJR Am J Roentgenol* 1990;155:143–151.

41. Spagnoli MV, Goldberg HI, Grossman RI Bilanink LT, Gomori JM, Hackney DB, Zimmerman RA. Intracranial meningiomas: high-field MR imaging. *Radiology* 1986;161:369–375.

42. Goldsher D, Litt AW, Pinto RS, Bannon KR, Kricheff II. Dural "tail'' associated with meningiomas on Gd-DTPA-enhanced MR images: characteristics, differential diagnostic value, and possible implications for treatment. *Radiology* 1990;176:447–450.

43. Valvassori GE, Garcia Morales F, Palacios E, Dobben GE. MR of the normal and abnormal internal auditory canal. *AJNR Am J Neuroradiol* 1989;9:115–119.

44. Weiner SN, Pearlstein AE, Eiber A. MR imaging of intracranial arachnoid cysts. *J Comput Assist Tomogr* 1987;11:236–241.

45. Tampieri D, Melanson D, Ethier R. MR imaging of epidermoid cysts. *AJNR Am J Neuroradiol* 1989; 10:351–356.

46. Smith AS, Benson JE, Blaser SI, Mizushima A, Tarr RW, Bellon EM. Diagnosis of ruptured intracranial dermoid cyst: value MR over CT. *AJNR Am J Neuroradiol* 1991;12:175–180.

47. Truwit CL, Barkovich AJ, Pathogenesis of intracranial lipoma: an MR study in 42 patients. *AJR Am J Roentgenol* 1990;155:855–864.

48. Kucharczyk W, Davis DO, Kelly WM, Sze G, Norman D, Newton TH. Pituitary adenomas: high resolution MR imaging at 1.5 T. *Radiology* 1986;161:761–765.

49. Newton DR, Dillon WP, Norman D, Newton TH, Wilson CB. Gd-DTPA-enhanced MR imaging of pituitary adenomas. *AJNR Am J Neuroradiol* 1989;10:949–954.

50. Freeman MP, Kessler RM, Allen JH, Price AC. Craniopharyngioma: CT and MR imaging in nine cases. *J Comput Assist Tomogr* 1987;11:810–814.

51. Kucharczyk W, Peck WW, Kelly WM, Norman D, Newton TH. Rathke cleft cysts: CT, MR imaging, and pathological features. *Radiology* 1987;165:491–495.

52. Bird CR, Drayer BP, Medina M, Rekate HL, Flom RA, Hodak JA. Gd-DTPA-enhanced MR imaging in pediatric patients after brain tumor resection. *Radiology* 1988;169:123–126.

53. Barkovich AJ, Norman D. Anomalies of the corpus callosum: correlation with further anomalies of the brain. *AJR Am J Roentgenol* 1988;151:171–179.

54. Barkovich AJ, Chuang SH, Norman D. MR of neuronal migration anomalies. *AJR Am J Roentgenol* 1988; 150:179–187.

55. Nyberg DA, Cyr DR, Mack LA, Fitzsimmons J, Hickok D, Mahoney BS. Dandy-Walker malformation prenatal sonographic diagnosis and its clinical significance. *J Ultrasound Med* 1988;7:65–71.

56. el Gammal T, Mark EK, Brooks BS. MR imaging of Chiari II malformation. *AJR Am J Roentgenol* 1988; 150:163–170.

3

Spine

INTRODUCTION

Magnetic resonance imaging (MRI) has replaced myelography and computed tomography (CT) as the modality of choice in spinal imaging in all but a few special circumstances. Largely this is the result of the noninvasive nature of MRI and its ability to cover large areas of the spine in short periods of time by using sagittal imaging planes. Also, MRI lacks the artifact from adjacent bone that plagues CT, and it has the ability to perform multiple sequences that enhance the detection of pathological conditions within the cord and thecal sac. T1-weighted sequences best demonstrate cord anatomy; T2-weighted or multiplanar gradient-recalled echo (MPGR) sequences give a myelographic effect, making the cerebrospinal fluid (CSF) appear bright and increasing the sensitivity for detection of intrinsic cord lesions (Fig. 1).

Spinal imaging is prone to artifacts resulting from motion, including CSF pulsations, cardiac activity, blood flow within adjacent vessels, and respiration and bowel peristaltic activity. These artifacts are most apparent on T2-weighted and MPGR sequences. The artifacts from CSF pulsations can be reduced by the use of flow compensation (gradient-moment nulling) on MPGR and standard T2-weighted sequences. Fast spin–echo (FSE) sequences in many circumstances are superior to MPGR or standard T2-weighted sequences in spinal imaging. The FSE technique in cervical and thoracic spinal imaging uses cardiac gating (which is easily performed with a peripheral lead on the patient's finger) to reduce the CSF pulsation artifact. The CSF pulsations tend not to be a significant factor in the lumbar spine; so gating is not required.

Respiratory, cardiovascular, and peristaltic motion can be markedly reduced by placing saturation pulse bands anterior to the spine. This helps eliminate the signal from moving anatomical parts anterior to the relatively stationary spine. The use of a surface coil positioned adjacent to the spine (the patient lies supine on top of the coil) also helps reduce some of the motion artifact because, as a result of the closer proximity of the coil, the signal from the spine makes a larger contribution to the image than does the signal emanating from moving anatomical parts at a greater distance anteriorly. The tradeoff is that an evaluation of the posterior paraspinous tissues is difficult with a surface coil because structures directly adjacent to the coil are intensely bright at the appropriate window and level settings for the spinal canal evaluation (Fig. 1).

When evaluating the spine for pathological disorders, it is important to develop a search pattern so that all pertinent anatomical parts will be examined. Beginning with the sagittal sequences, check the vertebral body alignment, bone marrow signal, and disc heights. Next, examine the cord for caliber or signal abnormalities from intrinsic lesions and for compression by extrinsic processes. Any abnormality should be confirmed on axial slices. The neural foramina should be examined to ensure the exiting nerves are unimpinged (fat should completely surround

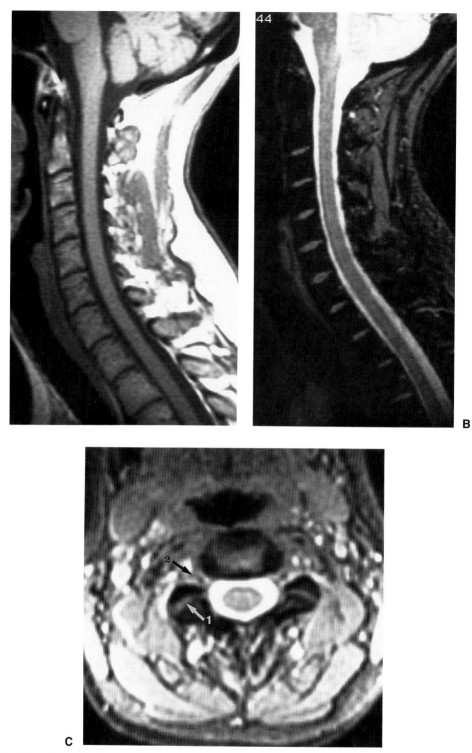

FIG. 1. Normal cervical and thoracic spine. **A:** A T1-weighted midline sagittal image demonstrates normal cervical vertebral bodies and intervening discs. The cervical spinal cord is normal in caliber and is homogeneously isointense with the brain. The surrounding CSF is hypointense. **B:** An MPGR sagittal cervical spine image has bright CSF surrounding the homogeneously hypointense spinal cord, which gives a myelographic effect. The vertebral bodies are hypointense because of a magnetic susceptibility artifact caused by the presence of calcium. **C:** An MPGR axial slice through the C2–3 disc space demonstrates hyperintense CSF surrounding the spinal cord. Normal facet joints (*1*) and neural foramina (*2*) are also seen.

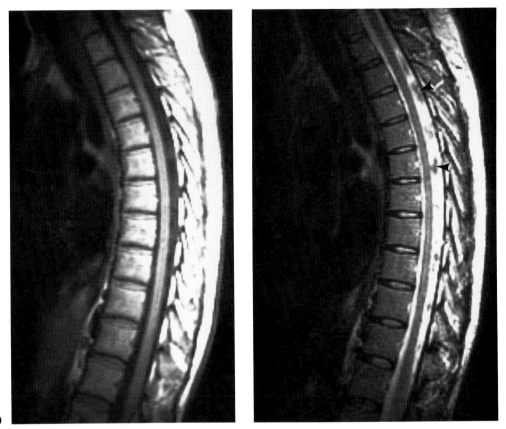

FIG. 1. *(continued)* **D:** A T1-weighted midline sagittal image of the thoracic spine demonstrates normal vertebral bodies and intervening disc spaces. The thoracic cord is normal in caliber and homogeneously intermediate in signal. The CSF is hypointense. Notice the posterior paraspinous tissues are poorly seen as a result of the relative hyperintensity of tissues directly adjacent to the surface coil. **E:** A T2-weighted, gated FSE sagittal image demonstrates decreased signal (compared with T1 weighting) from fatty marrow in the vertebral bodies. The disc nuclei and CSF are bright; the spinal cord is homogeneously hypointense. Multiple hypointense foci within the CSF posterior to the cord (*arrows*) are also seen. This does not represent a pathological condition but is artifactual, caused by CSF flow dynamics.

the nerves). The axial slices should then be examined level by level for spinal stenosis and narrowing of the neural foramina or lateral recesses. This may result from disc disease or bony abnormalities, including facet and ligamentous hypertrophy. The paraspinous soft tissues should be examined to exclude pathological conditions.

Formulating a differential diagnosis after an abnormality is found becomes easier if the lesion can be placed anatomically in one of three compartments: intramedullary (inside the spinal cord itself), intradural extramedullary (within the thecal sac but outside of the cord), and extradural (outside of the thecal sac but inside the spinal canal). Table 1 presents a useful differential diagnostic list for the more common abnormalities that occur in these compartments.

INTRAMEDULLARY ABNORMALITIES

In most cases, the spinal cord is best imaged with standard T1- and FSE T2-weighted sagittal sequences. T1- or T2-weighted axial scans

TABLE 1. *Differential diagnosis of spinal lesions by location*

Intramedullary
  Ependymoma
  Astrocytoma
  Syrinx
  Transverse myelitis
  Multiple sclerosis
  Myelomalacia (cord atrophy)
Intradural extramedullary
  Meningioma
  Neurofibroma
  Schwannoma
  Leptomeningeal metastasis (drop metastasis)
  Arachnoiditis
Extradural
  Disc
  Metastasis
  Hematoma
  Synovial cyst

can be performed through areas of questionable abnormality for further evaluation. The cord extends from the base of the skull to the conus medullaris, usually positioned between T-12 and L-2. Visually, the cord normally fills 50% to 75% of the anteroposterior diameter of the spinal canal. It is totally surrounded by CSF, which is contained by the meninges (thecal sac).

No abrupt caliber changes of the cord are normally seen. The intrinsic cord signal should be homogeneous, being intermediate in signal on T1-weighted images and somewhat hypointense on T2-weighted sequences (Fig. 1).

The most common spinal cord tumors are ependymomas and astrocytomas. Patients may present with back pain or bowel and bladder dysfunction. Ependymomas and astrocytomas have a similar appearance and cannot be reliably differentiated by MRI. Both cause cord widening or mass effect. They are hypo- or isointense with normal cord on T1 and hyperintense on T2. Both may contain cysts and hemorrhage with surrounding edema. Both show enhancement with gadolinium and have a predisposition for the thoracic cord, although a significant proportion of astrocytomas occur in the cervical cord. Ependymomas prefer the conus medullaris (Fig. 2) and filum terminale. Astrocytomas rarely involve the filum. Other intramedullary tumors, such as hemangioblastomas and metastases, are uncommon.

Both ependymomas and astrocytomas may be associated with a syrinx. A syrinx is a cavitary dilatation of the central cord filled with CSF and often containing septations (Fig. 3). Whenever a syrinx is encountered, gadolinium should be administered to evaluate for tumor enhancement. This can help differentiate a syrinx associated with a tumor from other causes of syringomyelia, such as trauma, arachnoiditis, and Chiari malformations.

Inflammatory processes can also cause focal spinal cord expansion and may mimic a neoplasm. Transverse myelitis is an example. Typically, this process is isointense to the normal cord on T1-weighted sequences and hyperintense on T2-weighted sequences. Mild gadolinium enhancement is also typical (Fig. 4). The prognosis is variable. The cord abnormality may totally resolve over weeks to become normal in appearance.

Multiple sclerosis is an inflammatory process that may be indistinguishable from transverse myelitis. It commonly involves the spinal cord and the brain. The cervical cord is affected more often than the thoracic cord. During active demyelination, the cord may be normal in caliber or focally swollen with an increased signal on T2-weighted images. Gadolinium enhancement is also seen (Fig. 5). Chronic plaques remain hyperintense on T2 but are nonenhancing and may result in focal cord atrophy. A similar atrophic appearance is seen with myelomalacia of any cause. Myelitis resulting from radiation therapy can also appear similar, except the adjacent vertebral bodies are generally hyperintense on T1-weighted images as a result of the fatty replacement of marrow within the radiation port.

INTRADURAL EXTRAMEDULLARY ABNORMALITIES

Intradural extramedullary abnormalities are contained within the spinal CSF spaces, anal-

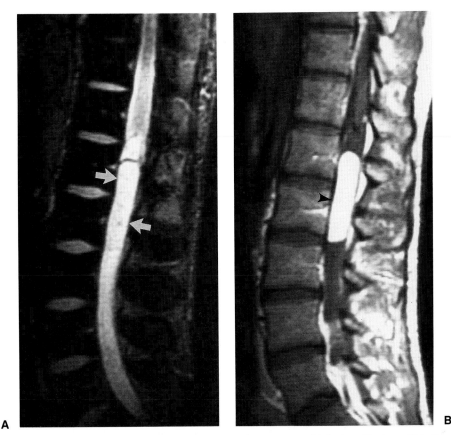

FIG. 2. Ependymoma. **A:** An MPGR sagittal image demonstrates a high signal lesion within the conus medullaris (*arrows*). **B:** A T1-weighted image with gadolinium shows a homogeneous, intensely enhancing, intramedullary tumor (*arrow*), widening the spinal cord.

ogous to extraaxial lesions of the brain. They can cause a mass effect, distorting the contour or deviating the adjacent spinal cord or nerve roots, but they arise outside of the cord itself. The presence of CSF surrounding much of the lesions surface helps differentiate intradural from extradural processes. Table 1 lists common abnormalities involving this space.

Neurofibroma, schwannoma, and meningioma are the major primary tumors arising within the intradural extramedullary space, although neurofibromas and schwannomas frequently (and meningiomas occasionally) also involve the extradural space. All three lesions are usually benign and may present with pain, sometimes radicular. If cord compression is present, bowel and bladder dysfunction may also be present. Meningiomas and schwanno-mas are usually solitary; neurofibromas are often multiple.

Neurofibroma and Schwannoma

Neurofibromas and schwannomas are nerve sheath tumors, arising along the nerve roots. They are usually multiple and associated with neurofibromatosis type 1 (peripheral form). Sagittal images may show scalloping of the vertebral bodies, corresponding to plain x-ray film findings, as a result of dural ectasia. The lesions themselves are best imaged in the coronal and axial projections. This best demonstrates expansion of the roots and neural foramina (Fig. 6). Neurofibromas are isointense or mildly hyperintense on T1-weighted sequences and markedly hyperintense on T2-

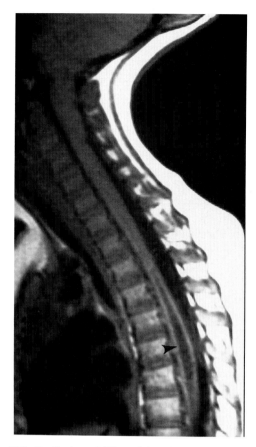

FIG. 3. Syrinx. A T1-weighted sagittal image demonstrates central cavitary dilation (*arrow*) of the upper thoracic cord. This syrinx was associated with an Arnold-Chiari II malformation.

weighted sequences. They typically enhance with gadolinium.

Meningioma

Most spinal meningiomas are thoracic in location. They are typically well circumscribed, attached to the dura, and nearly isointense with the spinal cord, although this is variable. The bright-signal-intensity CSF against the intermediate-signal-intensity mass on T2-weighted sequences optimizes detection. Similar to intracranial lesions, spinal meningiomas intensely enhance with gadolinium. Differentiation of meningiomas from solitary nerve sheath tumors (schwannoma) can be difficult

(Fig. 7). Treatment for a meningioma is surgical.

Leptomeningeal Metastasis

Most leptomeningeal metastases arise from primary brain tumors (see Chapter 2, Table 15) that spread along CSF pathways. Although drop metastasis can be found anywhere along the spinal cord, roots, and meninges, the most common location is posterior in the lumbosacral region, as a result of gravity. These lesions are often subtle and nearly isointense with CSF on T1- and T2-weighted sequences. Gadolinium enhancement is essential for lesion detection. Typically, T1-weighted sagittal images before and after gadolinium administration are needed to screen for leptomeningeal metastases (see Chapter 2, Fig. 33D). Axial postgadolinium images confirm an abnormality in regions of abnormal enhancement.

Arachnoiditis

Arachnoiditis most commonly results from previous surgery, but it may also be secondary to chemical irritation, hemorrhage, or infection. The MRI demonstrates thickening or clumping of nerve roots, arachnoid adhesions, or a soft tissue mass within the CSF space (Fig. 8). Arachnoiditis may be associated with a syrinx. Gadolinium should be administered in cases of a soft tissue mass or syrinx to evaluate for a tumor. Neoplastic processes usually enhance, whereas enhancement is more variable with arachnoiditis.

EXTRADURAL ABNORMALITIES

Like the intradural extramedullary lesions, extradural lesions also correspond to extraaxial processes, although they are positioned outside the meninges rather than within the CSF spaces. Neurological symptoms result from extrinsic compression of these lesions on the spinal cord or nerve roots. Table 1 lists common abnormalities involving this space.

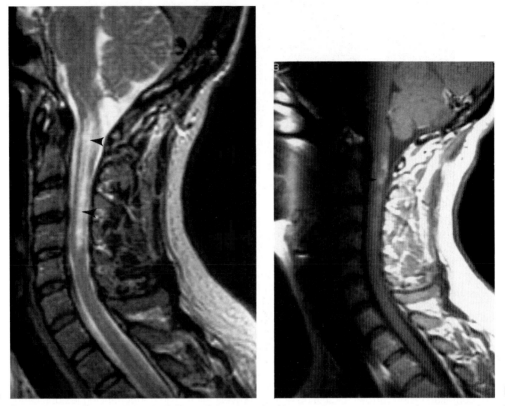

FIG. 4. Transverse myelitis. **A:** A T2-weighted sagittal image demonstrates an abnormal region of hyperintensity in the cervical cord (*arrows*). **B:** A T1-weighted image with gadolinium shows heterogeneous enhancement (*arrow*).

Tumor entering the extradural space usually arises from an adjacent vertebral body, either as a primary bone tumor or, more commonly, from the hematogenous spread of metastatic disease. Commonly seen metastases to vertebral bodies include breast, lung, and prostate cancer; lymphoma; and myeloma. T1-weighted sagittal images are best for detecting metastases to the bone because the normal bright fatty marrow is replaced by the lower-signal-intensity (water-containing) tumor cells (Fig. 9). When multiple vertebral bodies are involved, the level of confidence for the diagnosis of metastatic disease increases. However, when all vertebral bodies show a diffuse low signal intensity on the T1-weighted sequence, often, this is not a result of metastatic disease but of increased iron stores or increased red marrow (seen with chronic anemia). T2-weighted sagittal images may help differentiate these conditions because metastases commonly become hyperintense on T2 weighting, whereas red marrow and increased iron stores do not.

Metastatic disease may be associated with a vertebral body compression fracture. Acutely, these pathological fractures cannot be differentiated from osteoporotic fractures because both show low-signal-intensity marrow on T1-weighted images. Chronically (more than 6 weeks postfracture), however, even though diminished in height, the traumatic edema resolves, and the osteoporotic vertebral body will again show a normally bright fatty marrow signal, unlike a metastatic deposit, which remains low in signal intensity on T1 weighting.

Spinal metastases may present with pain, weakness, and at times, bowel and bladder dys-

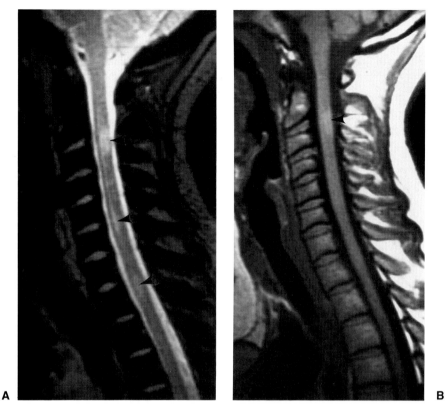

FIG. 5. Multiple sclerosis. **A:** An MPGR sagittal image demonstrates multiple hyperintense foci in the cervical spinal cord (*arrows*). **B:** A T1-weighted image with gadolinium shows enhancement of the most cephalad lesion (*arrow*), indicating active demyelination. The nonenhancing lesions caudally represent chronic plaques.

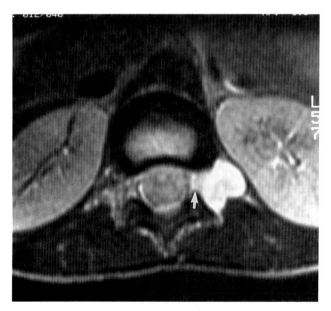

FIG. 6. Neurofibroma. A T2-weighted axial image of the upper lumbar spine demonstrates a hyperintense mass expanding the left neural foramen (*arrow*). It has both intradural and extradural components.

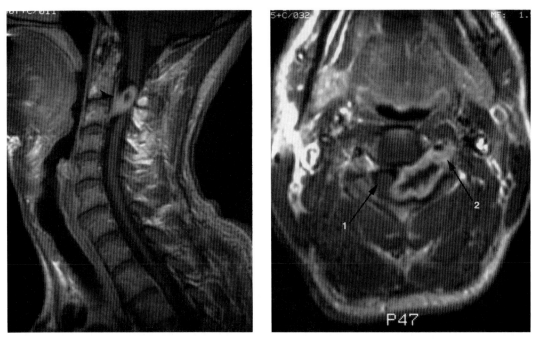

A

B

FIG. 7. Schwannoma. **A:** A T1-weighted sagittal image with gadolinium demonstrates an enhancing intradural mass with apparent attachment and extension along the dura anteriorly (*arrow*), suggesting meningioma. **B:** A T1-weighted axial image with gadolinium shows the enhancing mass to displace the spinal cord to the right (*1*) and expand the left C2–3 neural foramen (*2*). Foraminal expansion can occur with meningiomas or nerve sheath tumors. This tumor was a schwannoma.

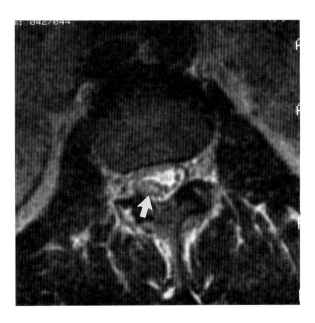

FIG. 8. Postoperative arachnoiditis. A T2-weighted FSE axial scan shows clumping of nerve roots in the thecal sac on the right (*arrow*).

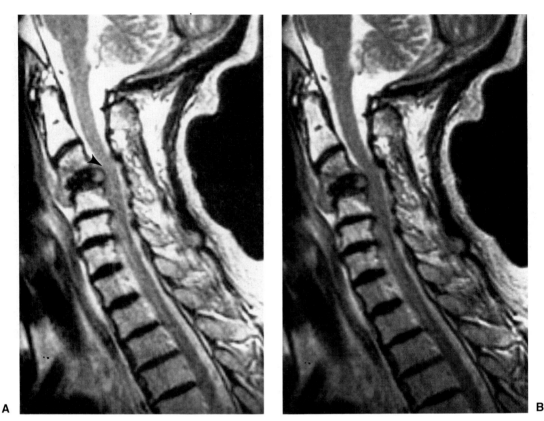

A   B

FIG. 9. Vertebral body metastasis (lung cancer). **A:** A T1-weighted sagittal image demonstrates a low-signal-intensity replacement of the normally bright marrow at C-3, C-4, and C-5 (posteriorly). A pathological fracture is present at C-4, causing extradural spinal cord compression (*arrow*). **B:** A T2-weighted FSE image shows signal increase in the sites of metastases, indicating increased water content (tumor cells).

function. A T1-weighted sagittal sequence is useful to exclude spinal cord compression by an extradural mass. Because the mass usually arises from a vertebral body, it is most often centered at the vertebral body rather than at a disc space. When cord compression occurs, the CSF space is obliterated, and the cord contour is deformed by the mass (Fig. 9). This is best confirmed by axial T1-weighted slices through the area of abnormality. Gadolinium is usually unnecessary but, occasionally, is helpful in defining the tumor margins.

An abnormal low signal within two adjacent vertebral bodies on a T1-weighted sequence, with narrowing of the intervening disc and in the presence of a paraspinous mass, suggests discitis rather than metastasis (Fig. 10). The paraspinous inflammatory mass is usually centered at the disc space rather than at a vertebral body. Degenerative discogenic vertebral sclerosis can appear to be similar, except the intervening degenerative disc has a low signal intensity on T2 weighting and no paraspinous mass is associated. Gadolinium administration is useful in defining the inflammatory process in cases of infectious discitis.

DEGENERATIVE DISEASE IN THE CERVICAL AND THORACIC SPINES

When evaluating the cervical and thoracic spines for spondylosis and disc disease, T1- and T2-weighted FSE sagittal sequences are indicated. In the cervical spine, an MPGR axial

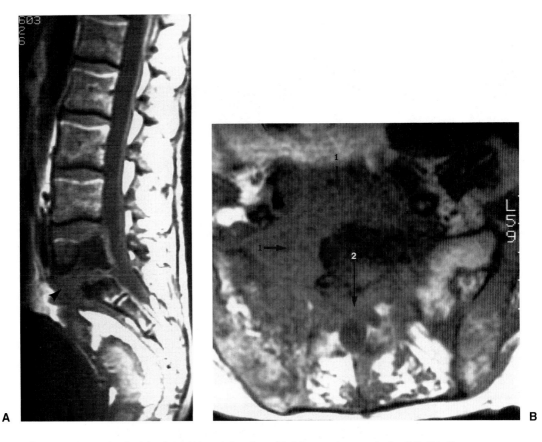

FIG. 10. Infectious discitis. **A:** A T1-weighted sagittal image demonstrates L5–S1 disc space narrowing, with abnormal low-signal-intensity marrow in the adjacent vertebral bodies. An anterior soft tissue mass is present, centered at the disc space (*arrow*). **B:** A T1-weighted axial slice at L5–S1 shows extension of the inflammation into the anterior and right aspect of the sacrum (*1*) and into the spinal canal (extradural space) to abut the thecal sac (*2*).

sequence is also necessary. The axial sequence can be performed as a two-dimensional multiplanar or three-dimensional volumetric scan. Although the three-dimensional volume study yields thinner slices, it suffers in its signal-to-noise ratio. The two-dimensional multiplanar sequence is adequate in most circumstances. If axial slices are needed along the thoracic spine, T1- or T2-weighted FSE sequences may be helpful. Axial MPGR sequences are often disappointing in the thoracic spine because of the presence of CSF pulsation and vascular flow artifacts.

The most common cause of spinal stenosis and neuroforaminal narrowing in the cervical and thoracic spines is the formation of osteo-phytes (spondylosis). Disc herniations are less common, especially in the thoracic spine. An osteophyte projecting into the central canal, centered at a cervical disc space, is sometimes called "hard disc" formation. Osteophytes tend to be isointense with bone on T1- and T2-weighted images and become dark on MPGR sequences. This helps differentiate an osteophyte from an acute disc herniation, which is bright on T2 and MPGR sequences (Fig. 11).

The spinal cord should be completely surrounded by CSF. When the CSF space is significantly reduced or effaced (usually anteriorly and posteriorly), spinal stenosis is present. When focal cord contour deformity is seen, cord compression is present. The diagnosis of

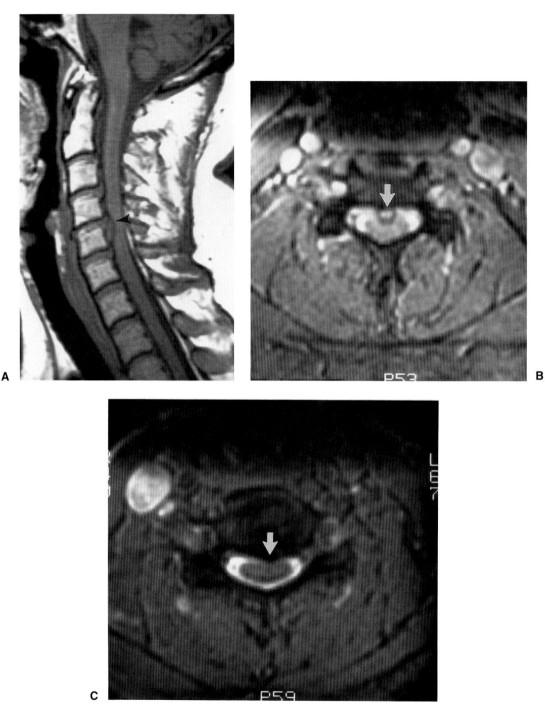

FIG. 11. Cervical disc herniation *versus* osteophytic formation. **A:** In a 45-year-old woman, a T1-weighted sagittal image demonstrates disc space narrowing at C3–4 and C4–5. The tissue is isointense with the disc and is seen extending posteriorly into the extradural space of the spinal canal (*arrow*). **B:** In the same patient, the MPGR axial image at C4–5 shows hyperintense material centrally in the anterior spinal canal (*arrow*), causing mild cord compression. This appearance is characteristic of an extruded (herniated) disc. **C:** An MPGR axial image at C5–6 in a 49-year-old woman, showing mild spinal stenosis as a result of a hypointense osteophyte projecting into the spinal canal (*arrow*).

thoracic cord compression as a result of disc herniation is similar to that in the cervical spine. However, because of the inherently small thoracic canal dimensions, a small disc or osteophyte may result in cord compression (Fig. 12).

Neural foraminal narrowing is a subjective finding and is best evaluated on axial sequences (Fig. 13). The nonspin–echo MPGR images may overestimate the degree of narrowing in the presence of osteophytes as a result of magnetic susceptibility artifact (blooming).

DEGENERATIVE DISEASE IN THE LUMBAR SPINE

An evaluation of lumbosacral disc disease is generally performed with T2-weighted images in both the sagittal and axial planes. The FSE images are preferred because of the increase in T2 weighting with the reduced imaging time. A T1-weighted sagittal sequence to evaluate the bone marrow should be added.

The normal disc appears intermediate in signal intensity on T1-weighted sequences and increased in signal on T2-weighted images. An axial slice through a normal disc level demonstrates a symmetric disc contour without a focal bulge or thecal sac effacement. Exiting nerve roots are seen within the neural foramina surrounded by perineural fat. With age and as degeneration occurs, disc height is lost, and the disc becomes increasingly desiccated, having a low signal intensity on T2-weighted images (Fig. 14).

When disc material extends beyond the adjacent vertebral bodies, spinal stenosis with impingement on the thecal sac may occur. Nar-

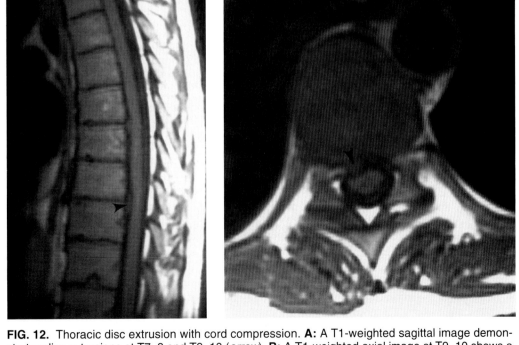

A   B

FIG. 12. Thoracic disc extrusion with cord compression. **A:** A T1-weighted sagittal image demonstrates disc extrusions at T7–8 and T9–10 (*arrow*). **B:** A T1-weighted axial image at T9–10 shows a right paracentral disc extrusion (*arrow*) deforming the contour of the spinal cord (cord compression).

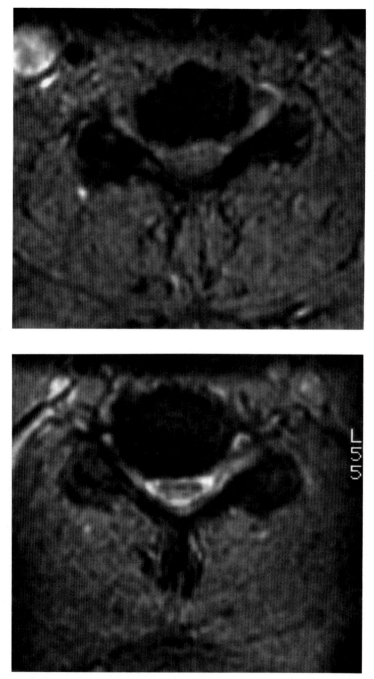

A

B

FIG. 13. Cervical neural foraminal narrowing. The MPGR axial images through the lower cervical disc levels demonstrate spondylitic (osteophytic) changes. **A:** Subjectively, moderate right and mild left foraminal narrowing is present, with spinal canal stenosis (bright CSF does not surround the cord). **B:** Severe right foraminal stenosis is present. The left neural foramen is normal.

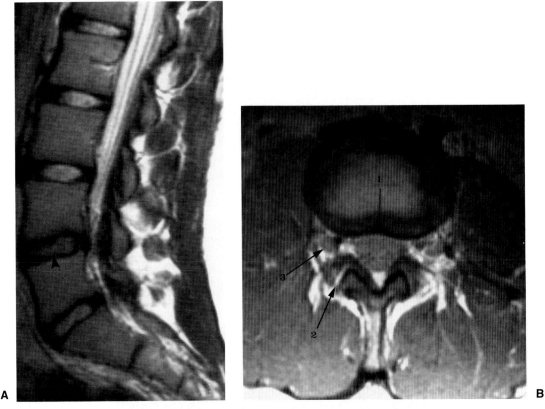

FIG. 14. Normal disc level and disc desiccation. **A:** A T2-weighted sagittal image demonstrates multiple normal disc levels with a hyperintense signal. Disc desiccation from degeneration is seen at L4–5, resulting in hypointensity (*arrow*). **B:** A normal axial proton density FSE image at L3–4 shows symmetric disc contour abutting the thecal sac (*1*), normal facet joints (*2*), and exiting nerves (*3*) surrounded by perineural fat within the neural foramina.

rowing of the lateral recesses or neural foramina may also occur. The neural foramina are positioned along the cephalad aspect of the disc space in the lumbar spine. Nerve roots in the lumbar spine exit the foramina beneath the corresponding pedicle of the same level (i.e., the L-4 nerve root exits beneath the L-4 pedicle). Narrowing of the neural foramen or lateral recess causes radicular symptoms along that particular nerve's distribution (i.e., L-4 in this example). Impingement on the thecal sac by disc disease typically causes radicular symptoms at the next root level (i.e., canal impingement by a L4–5 disc causes L-5 symptoms.) This is because the site of thecal sac impingement is typically caudal to the level of the corresponding neural foramina.

Disc disease is diagnosed and classified morphologically on MRI in the same way as by CT, i.e., annular bulge, protrusion, extrusion, or free fragment (Fig. 15). Depending on the severity of the mass effect from the disc disease and the intrinsic dimensions of the spinal canal, significant stenosis may occur.

A relatively symmetrically bulging disc that extends beyond the margins of the adjacent vertebral bodies is an annular bulge. An asymmetric, broad-based, focal disc bulge is called a disc protrusion. This may project posteriorly, causing spinal stenosis, or laterally, causing isolated neural foraminal narrowing. A focal mass of disc material that, instead of causing a broad bulge, causes focal alteration in the expected disc contour is called an extrusion. It

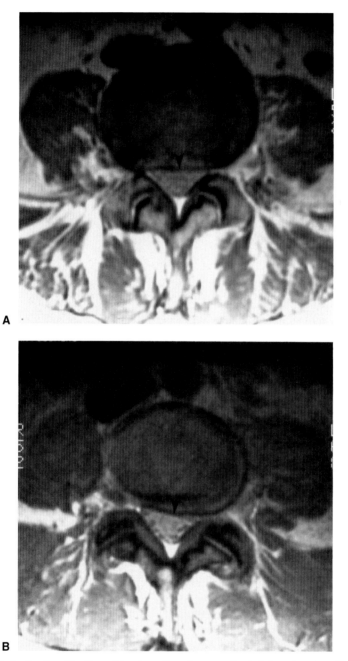

FIG. 15. Morphologic classification of lumbar disc disease. **A:** Axial proton density images show a broad annular disc bulge, which causes mild linear flattening of the thecal sac (*arrow*). **B:** Disc protrusion with the asymmetrically bulging disc (*arrow*) deforming the left aspect of the thecal sac and narrowing the left neural foramen.

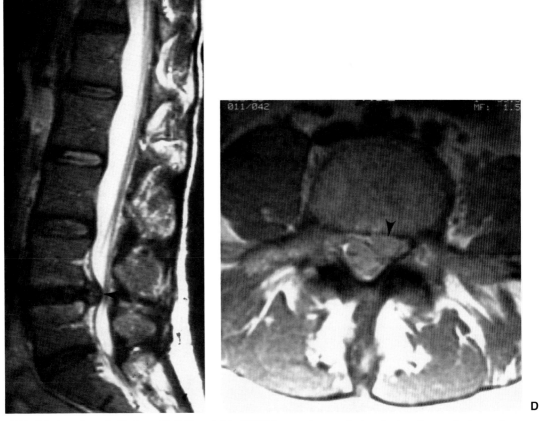

C   D

FIG. 15. *(continued)* **C:** A sagittal T2-weighted FSE image demonstrates desiccation and a large disc extrusion (*arrow*) at L4–5. **D:** An axial proton density FSE image in another patient shows a disc extrusion. It fills the left lateral recess (*arrow*) and deforms the left aspect of the thecal sac at the vertebral body level directly cephalad to the parent disc.

is this abnormality that is commonly referred to as disc herniation. When a mass of disc material migrates away from the donor disc, so that it is no longer in continuity, it is called a free fragment.

The grading of spinal stenosis is somewhat subjective, but it is often judged as mild, moderate, or severe, depending on the degree of central canal diameter narrowing and the distortion of the thecal sac (Fig. 16). Several factors may contribute to central canal stenosis (and neural foraminal narrowing). These include congenital stenosis, resulting from short pedicles, disc disease, and facet and ligamentum flavum hypertrophy. Anteriorly, the axial contours of the thecal sac at L1–2, L2–3, and L3–4 are typically convex (Fig. 14B). When flattening or a concavity is present, spinal steno-

sis should be considered. Axial flattening of the anterior contour at L4–5 and L5–S1 may occur normally, but in general, a concave thecal sac contour is abnormal. Effacement of the fat planes that normally surround portions of the thecal sac is another circumstance in which spinal stenosis should be considered.

A synovial cyst is an occasional cause of thecal sac compression. It arises at a facet joint, probably from degeneration. Generally, it is isointense or slightly hyperintense to CSF on T1 and T2 weighting (Fig. 17).

POSTOPERATIVE LUMBAR SPINE

When low-back pain or radicular pain persists or recurs after surgery, the imager may be called on to determine if recurrent disc disease

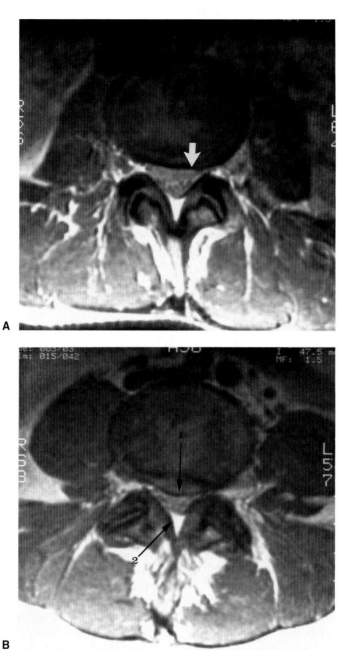

FIG. 16. Subjective grading of spinal stenosis using axial proton density FSE images. **A:** Mild spinal stenosis. Left-sided disc protrusion (*arrow*) causes mild thecal sac deformity and neural foraminal narrowing. Mild ligamentum flavum hypertrophy is also seen. **B:** Moderate spinal stenosis. Broad central disc protrusion (*1*) causes moderate thecal sac deformity. Mild to moderate facet and ligamentum flavum hypertrophy also contribute to the overall reduction in the size of the spinal canal.

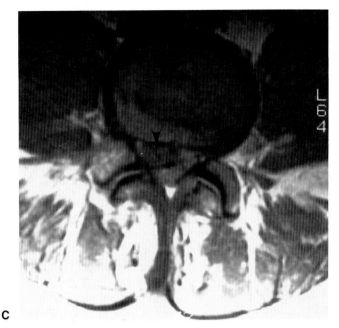

C

FIG. 16. *(continued)* **C:** Severe spinal stenosis. A large right paracentral disc extrusion (*arrow*) causes marked thecal sac deformity.

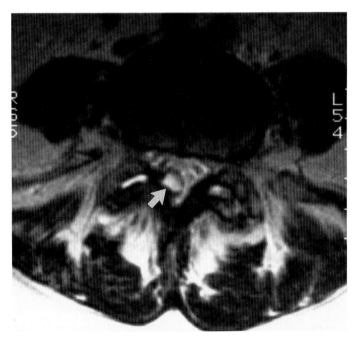

FIG. 17. Synovial cyst. An axial T2-weighted FSE image at L4–5 shows a hyperintense, fluid-filled cyst (*arrow*) arising from the right facet joint, causing deformity on the adjacent thecal sac.

is present. The postoperative examination needs to be tailored so that the ability to differentiate recurrent disc herniation from postoperative scarring is maximized. This is important because, in general, surgical removal of recurrent disc material may relieve the symptoms, whereas reoperating on scar tissue does not. Imaging is best done by performing T1-weighted sagittal and axial sequences pre- and post-gadolinium administration. Scar tissue will generally show heterogeneous enhancement (Fig. 18), whereas in general, disc material does not enhance. Gadolinium should always be used for the evaluation of the postoperative spine. It is also useful in the evaluation of infectious complications.

CONGENITAL SPINAL ABNORMALITIES

The neural groove forms from the migration of ectodermal cells and closes to become the neural tube by about 4 weeks of gestation (neurulation). Closure begins in the cervical region and proceeds both cranially and caudally. The spinal cord forms within the neural tube. Further elongation and differentiation proceeds caudally, eventually forming the distal conus medullaris and filum terminale (canalization and retrogressive differentiation). The development of vertebral bodies also occurs during this stage of gestation. Congenital anomalies of the spine are a result of an abnormality in one or more steps of the developmental process.

When imaging congenital spinal abnormalities, it is generally sufficient to acquire T1-weighted sagittal and axial sequences through the region of interest. Additional T2-weighted and gradient-recalled echo sequences may be helpful in special circumstances, such as the evaluation of tumors or confirming the presence of calcification.

Spinal dysraphism, which results from incomplete closure of the neural tube, may be present as a myelomeningocele in which the neural elements are externalized without overlying skin. Preoperative imaging of the spine is usually unnecessary. In general, postopera-

tive imaging of the spine is needed only when the patient's functioning deteriorates and postoperative complications are sought. These complications include retethering of the cord by scar, the inclusion of material (resulting in an epidermoid or lipoma), and cord infarction.

Occult spinal dysraphisms are skin-covered defects of neural tube closure, such as lipomyeloceles, lipomyelomeningoceles, intradural lipomas (rare), and dorsal dermal sinuses. Like myelomeningoceles, lipomyelomeningoceles are always associated with a tethered cord. Even though the conus medullaris normally ascends during childhood, in general, it should always be positioned cephalad to the L-3 level. When the conus is positioned at L-3 or below, a tethered cord should be strongly considered. Symptoms of a tethered cord include club feet, bladder dysfunction, and leg pain. Although tethered cords are often diagnosed within the first year of life, they sometimes remain asymptomatic until discovered in adulthood.

Lipomyeloceles and lipomyelomeningoceles generally occur in the lumbar region. The distal malformed spinal cord (placode) terminates into a lipoma that tethers it to the body wall (Fig. 19). A fibrolipoma of the filum terminale is generally an asymptomatic, incidental finding (Fig. 20.) The lipomatous tissues associated with these lesions is easily visualized because of their high signal on T1-weighted images.

When focal failure of neural ectoderm separation from superficial ectoderm occurs during neural tube closure, a dorsal dermal sinus results. This sinus extends variable distances into the body wall from a midline dimple in the skin surface. It may enter the spinal canal and dura, usually in the lumbosacral region. The dermal sinus tract ends in a dermoid or epidermoid in a majority of cases. The symptoms include infection or compression by an associated dermoid or epidermoid (Fig. 21). Dermoids contain fat and are readily detectable on T1-weighted images. Epidermoids may be isointense to the CSF and difficult to see.

Diastematomyelia is a sagittal division of the spinal cord that results from splitting of the notochord during cell migration. The two hemi-

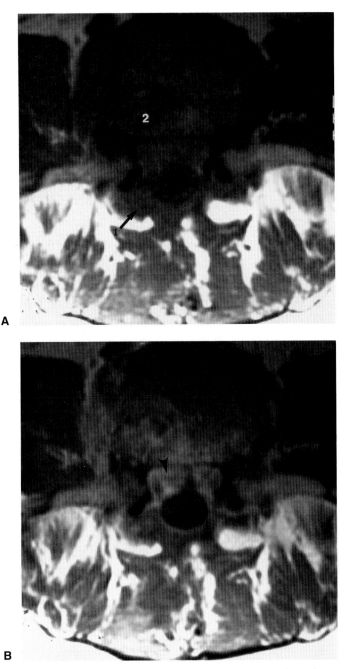

FIG. 18. Postoperative scar. Axial T1-weighted images were performed to rule out recurrent disc disease. **A:** A laminectomy defect is present (*1*). Hypointense material fills the spinal canal (*2*) abutting the thecal sac. **B:** After gadolinium administration, there is diffuse enhancement (increased signal) of the material (scar) within the spinal canal (*arrow*). Only the thecal sac and transversing nerve roots remain hypointense. Nonenhancing material (disc) is not seen within the spinal canal.

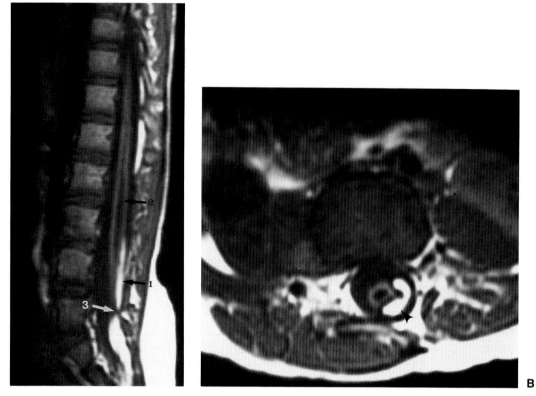

A   B

FIG. 19. Occult spinal dysraphism. Lipomyelocele in an 8-year-old girl. **A:** A T1-weighted sagittal image demonstrates a lipoma along the posterior aspect of the spinal cord (*1*), causing cord tethering. A syrinx is present within the distal cord (*2*). The conus medullaris (*3*) is positioned at L-5. **B:** An axial T1-weighted image demonstrates the lipoma (high signal intensity) adjacent to the spinal cord (*arrow*). The low-signal-intensity central cord syrinx is also confirmed.

cords often reunite distal to the cleft. A bony spur or fibrous septum may be seen in the cleft, but it is present in less than one-half of the cases (Fig. 22). Most cases are associated with vertebral body abnormalities. The symptoms are similar to those of a tethered cord.

BIBLIOGRAPHY

Books

1. Atlas SW. *Magnetic resonance imaging of the brain and spine.* New York: Raven Press; 1991.
2. Barkovich AJ. *Pediatrics neuroimaging.* New York: Raven Press; 1990.

Journals

1. Karnaze MG, Gado MH, Sartor KJ, Hodges J. Comparison of MR and CT myelography in imaging of the cervical and thoracic spine. *AJR Am J Roentgenol* 1988;150:397–403.
2. Hyman RA, Gorey MT. Imaging strategies for MR of the spine. *Radiol Clin North Am* 1988;26:505–533.
3. Zimmerman RA, Bilaniuk LT. Imaging of tumors of the spinal canal and cord. *Radiol Clin North Am* 1988;26:965–1007.
4. Parizel PM, Balerieux D, Rodesch G, et al. Gd-DTPA enhanced MR imaging of spinal tumors. *AJR Am J Roentgenol* 1989;152:1087–1096.
5. Slasky BS, Bydder GM, Niendorf HP, Young IR. MR imaging with gadolinium-DTPA in differentiation of tumor, syrinx and cyst of the spinal cord. *J Comput Assist Tomogr* 1987;11:845–850.
6. Barakos JA, Mark AS, Dillon WP, Norman D. MR imaging of acute transverse myelitis and AIDS myelopathy. *J Comput Assist Tomogr* 1990;14:45–50.

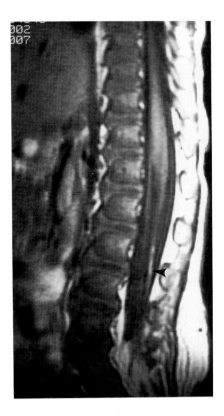

FIG. 20. Fibrolipoma of the filum terminale. A T1-weighted sagittal image demonstrates a thickened hyperintense filum terminale (*arrow*).

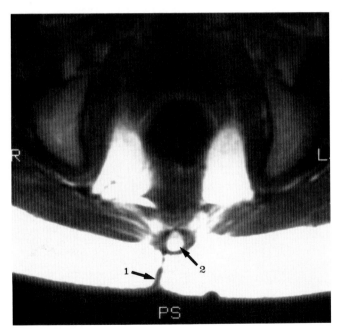

FIG. 21. Dorsal dermal sinus. A T1-weighted sagittal image in a 5-year-old girl demonstrates a low-signal-intensity sinus tract (*1*) extending from the skin surface to a high-signal-intensity mass (dermoid, *2*).

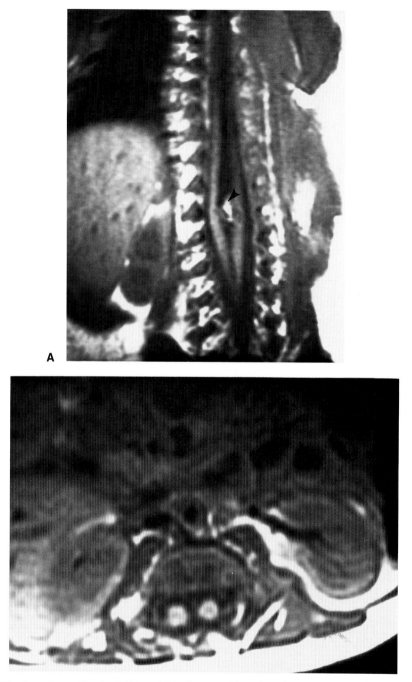

FIG. 22. Diastematomyelia. **A:** A T1-weighted coronal imaging demonstrates a bony spur (*arrow*) separating two hemicords. **B:** An axial T1-weighted image confirms the presence of two hemicords.

7. Maravilla KR, Weinreb JC, Suss R, Nunnally RL. Magnetic resonance demonstration of multiple sclerosis plaques in the cervical cord. *AJR Am J Roentgenol* 1985;144:381–385.

8. Larsson EM, Holtas S, Nilsson O. Gd-DTPA enhanced MR of suspected spinal multiple sclerosis. *AJNR Am J Neuroradiol* 1989;10:1071–1076.

9. Quencer RM, Sheldon JJ, Post MJ, Diaz RD, Montalvo BM, Green BA, Eismont FJ. MR of the chronically injured cervical spinal cord. *AJR Am J Roentgenol* 1986;147:125–132.

10. Zweig G, Russell EJ. Radiation myelopathy of the cervical spinal cord: MR findings. *AJNR Am J Neuroradiol* 1990;11:1188–1190.

11. Stevens SK, Moore SG, Kaplan ID. Early and late bone marrow changes after irradiation: MR evaluation. *AJR Am J Roentgenol* 1990;154:745–750.

12. Scotti G, Scialfa G, Colombo N, Landoni L. MR imaging of intradural extramedullary tumors of the cervical spine. *J Comput Assist Tomogr* 1985;9:1037–1041.

13. Burk DL Jr, Brumberg JA, Kanal E, Latchaw RE, Wolf GL. Spinal and paraspinal neurofibromatosis: surface coil MR imaging at 1.5 T. *Radiology* 1987;162:797–801.

14. Blews DE, Wang H, Kumar AJ, Robb PA, Phillips PC, Bryan RN. Intradural spinal metastases in pediatric patients with primary intracranial neoplasms: Gd-DTPA enhanced MR vs. CT myelography. *J Comput Assist Tomogr* 1990;14:730–735.

15. Johnson CE, Sze G. Benign lumbar arachnoiditis: MR imaging with gadopentatate dimeglumine. *AJR Am J Roentgenol* 1990;155:873–880.

16. Daffner RH, Lupetin AR, Dash N, Zeeb ZL, Sefczek RJ, Shapiro RL. MRI in the detection of malignant infiltration of bone marrow. *AJR Am J Roentgenol* 1986;146:353–358.

17. Smith SR, Williams CE, Davies JM, Edwards RH. Bone marrow disorders: characterization with quantitative MR imaging. *Radiology* 1989;172:805–810.

18. Carmody RF, Yang PJ, Seely GW, Seeger JF, Unger EC, Johnson JE. Spinal cord compression due to metastatic disease: diagnosis with MR versus myelography. *Radiology* 1989;173:225–229.

19. Post MJ, Sze G, Quencer RM, Eismont FJ, Green BA, Gahbauer H. Gadolinium enhanced MR in spinal infection. *J Comput Assist Tomogr* 1990;14:721–729.

20. Jahnke RW, Hart BL. Cervical stenosis, spondylosis, and herniated disc disease. *Radiol Clin North Am* 1991;29:777–791.

21. Rosenbloom SA. Thoracic disc disease and stenosis. *Radiol Clin North Am* 1991;29:765–775.

22. Gaskill MF, Lukin R, Wiot JG. Lumbar disc disease and stenosis. *Radiol Clin North Am* 1991;29:753–764.

23. Hueftle MG, Modic MT, Ross JS, et al. Lumbar spine: postoperative MR imaging with Gd-DTPA. *Radiology* 1988;167:817–824.

24. Altman NR, Altman DH. MR imaging of spinal dysraphism. *AJNR Am J Neuroradiol* 1987;8:533–538.

25. Raghavan N, Barkovich AJ, Edwards M, Norman D. MR imaging in the tethered spinal cord syndrome. *AJR Am J Roentgenol* 1989;152:843–852.

26. Barkovich AJ, Edwards M, Cogen PH. MR evaluation of spinal dermoid sinus tracts in children. *AJNR Am J Neuroradiol* 1991;12:123–124.

4

Head and Neck

ORBITS

In most circumstances, the axial and coronal planes are best for orbital imaging with magnetic resonance imaging (MRI). Standard T1-weighted and fast spin–echo (FSE) T2-weighted sequences may be used. However, for an evaluation of a tumor or inflammation, T1-weighted sequences with fat saturation pre- and postgadolinium enhancement are often essential. The use of fat saturation is the key to evaluating for contrast enhancement; otherwise, the abundant signal from orbital fat may completely obscure the bright T1 signal from the gadolinium.

The orbital anatomy can be divided into several compartments, which are anatomically important and help in formulating differential diagnoses. The extraocular muscles extend from the globe toward the orbital apex, surrounding the orbital contents in the shape of a cone. All the orbital contents within this muscular cone are within the intraconal space. Those outside the muscular cone, but inside the surrounding periosteum, are within the extraconal space. A connective tissue extension of the periosteum anterior to the intraocular muscles attaches to the eyelids, anatomically separating the orbit into anterior preseptal and posterior postseptal spaces (Fig. 1). This anatomic barrier is important because it acts to limit the spread of infection from one compartment to the other.

The lacrimal gland is positioned superolaterally in the preseptal space. The tears are drained by the lacrimal duct, positioned in the preseptal space inferomedially. The preseptal space is extraconal, whereas the postseptal space contains both intra- and extraconal compartments. When considering orbital pathological conditions, whether by computed tomography (CT) or MRI, it is useful to formulate a differential diagnosis based on the location of the lesion within the orbit. Differential diagnostic possibilities will be presented, and although these limited lists still tend to be lengthy, many lesions are relatively rare. Only selected disorders will be individually discussed.

Table 1 lists the major diagnostic possibilities for a mass of the globe. Melanomas and orbital metastases are generally unilateral, occur in adults, and enhance with gadolinium. As a result of the T1 and T2 shortening by melanin, melanomas (in the absence of hemorrhage) are often bright on T1- and dark on T2-weighted sequences. This helps differentiate them from other masses, such as metastases, which generally are dark on T1 and bright on T2 (Fig. 2). Retinoblastomas occur in childhood, are bilateral one-third of the time, enhance with gadolinium, and typically, contain calcification. Because calcification may be the dominant feature, CT is preferred over MRI for

TABLE 1. *Differential diagnosis of globe masses*

Melanoma
Metastases
Retinoblastoma
Benign masses (e.g., hemangioma or hamartoma, rare)

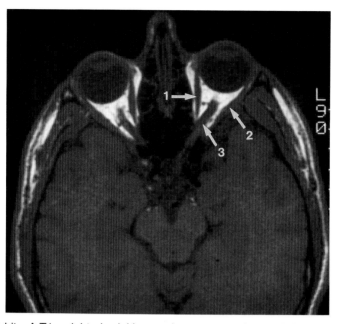

FIG. 1 Normal orbits. A T1-weighted axial image demonstrates the medial (*1*) and lateral (*2*) rectus muscles. The outer aspect of the rectus muscles separates the intraconal from the extraconal space. The optic nerves (*3*) are seen exiting at the orbital apices.

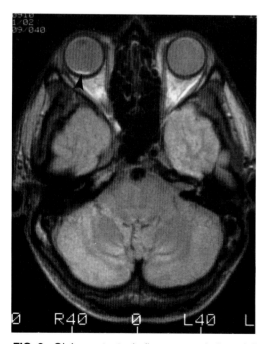

FIG. 2. Globe metastasis (lung cancer). An axial proton density image demonstrates a subtle, hyperintense retinal mass (*arrow*) in the right orbit.

detection of these lesions. When evaluating a patient with a primary orbital malignant neoplasm, it is important to understand that metastases from the orbit will be hematogenous because the orbit has no lymphatic drainage.

The pre- and postseptal spaces may be affected by a number of abnormalities, some of which are listed in Tables 2 to 6. Most inflammatory and neoplastic processes encountered will be hypointense on T1 and hyperintense on T2 weighting, and they will enhance with gadolinium. This makes differentiation between tumors and inflammatory processes difficult. The clinical history is often helpful. Pseudotumor, which is a benign inflammatory process that results in a focal or diffuse lymphocytic infiltration, may appear identical to lymphoma. They both can cause soft tissue swelling, mass infiltration into orbital fat, thickening of extraocular muscles, and enlargement of the lacrimal gland (Fig. 3). Pseudotumor is typically of rapid onset and painful, and it responds rapidly to corticosteroid therapy. Lymphoma

TABLE 2. *Differential diagnosis of abnormalities involving the preseptal space*

Cellulitis
Pseudotumor
Lymphoma
Metastasis
Dermoid
Lymphangioma
Lacrimal gland tumor or inflammatory process

TABLE 3. *Differential diagnosis of lacrimal gland enlargement*

Primary lacrimal tumor (benign or malignant, similar
  to minor salivary gland histology)
Lymphoma
Metastasis
Pseudotumor (pseudolymphoma)
Dacryoadenitis
Dermoid cyst
Sjögren's disease

TABLE 4. *Differential diagnosis of intraconal abnormalities*

Hemangioma
Pseudotumor (pseudolymphoma)
Lymphoma
Metastasis
Process causing thickening of extraocular
  musculature
Optic nerve or sheath lesions

TABLE 5. *Differential diagnosis of extraocular muscle thickening*

Graves's disease (thyroid ophthalmopathy)
Pseudotumor
Lymphoma
Metastasis
Venous congestion
Rhabdomyosarcoma

TABLE 6. *Differential diagnosis of optic nerve or sheath lesions*

Optic nerve glioma
Meningioma
Optic neuritis
Pseudotumor
Pseudolymphoma
Lymphoma
Graves's disease

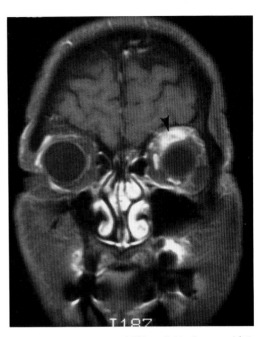

FIG. 3. Pseudotumor. A T1-weighted coronal fat-saturated sequence with gadolinium demonstrates a markedly thickened, enhancing (hyperintense) superior rectus muscle on the left (*arrow*).

typically is of slower onset and painless. Cellulitis can also appear similar, but it usually arises from adjacent, visualizable sinus disease (Fig. 4). Although often limited to the preseptal space, the extraconal spread of infection into the posterior orbit and venous extension (causing cavernous sinus thrombosis) are possible complications of cellulitis.

Focal masses can occur anywhere in the preseptal space, but they favor the superolateral aspect in the region of the lacrimal gland. Most of these lesions have similar signal characteristics on MRI, yielding low specificity. One notable exception is an orbital dermoid. Because this lesion contains fat it will be isointense to the retroglobar or subcutaneous fat. Loss of lesion signal on a fat-saturated sequence is confirmatory. Hemorrhagic lesions typically remain hyperintense on T1 weighting with fat saturation (Fig. 5).

Cavernous hemangiomas are common vascular tumors of the orbit. They are usually intraconal but may arise or extend extraconally. MRI demonstrates a well-defined mass whose

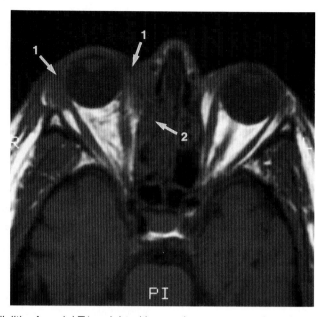

FIG. 4. Orbital cellulitis. An axial T1-weighted image demonstrates a low-signal-intensity inflammatory mass filling the orbital preseptal space on the right (*1*). The cellulitis arose from ethmoid sinusitis (*2*). Notice that the infection is effectively confined within the preseptal space.

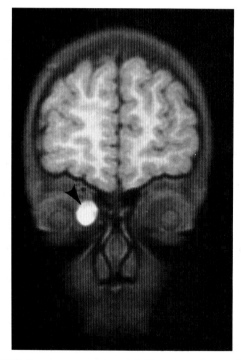

FIG. 5. Hemorrhagic orbital lymphangioma. A coronal T1-weighted fat-saturated sequence demonstrates a rounded, hyperintense mass in the superomedial orbit (*arrow*) on the right.

signal intensity is primarily low (isointense with muscle) on T1, and hyperintense on T2 weighting (Fig. 6).

Thickening of the extraocular muscles can result from a number of processes, some of the more common ones are listed in Table 5. Essentially all these lesions are isointense with muscle on T1 weighting. Metastases (occur in adults) and rhabdomyosarcomas (occur in children) are typically hyperintense on T2-weighted sequences (Fig. 7). The more common abnormalities, including Graves's disease, pseudotumor, and lymphoma, are often isointense or nearly isointense to muscle on T2, making their differentiation more difficult. Graves's disease is usually bilateral, involving multiple extraocular muscles, and seldom involves the lateral rectus alone (Fig. 8). Pseudotumor is usually unilateral and may involve any muscle or combination of muscles. Lymphomatous involvement of the extraocular muscles is more difficult to differentiate, but it is a much less common abnormality.

Enlargement of the optic nerve sheath can be a result of numerous processes (Table 6).

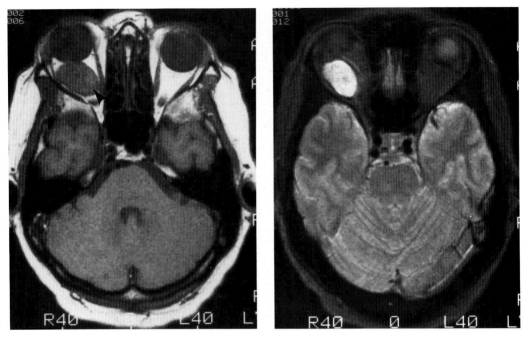

FIG. 6. Orbital hemangioma. **A:** A T1-weighted axial image demonstrates a well-defined, oval, hypointense, intraconal mass (*arrow*) situated between the optic nerve and lateral rectus muscle. **B:** A T2-weighted sequence shows the mass to be hyperintense.

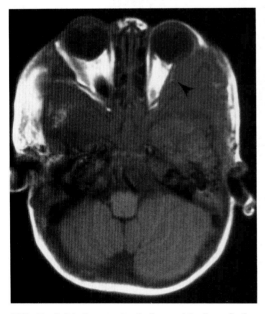

FIG. 7. Orbital metastasis (neuroblastoma). An axial T1-weighted image demonstrates a low-signal-intensity tumor invading the base of the skull anteriorly. The tumor has extended into the lateral aspect of the orbit on the right, invading and thickening the lateral rectus muscle (*arrow*).

Optic nerve gliomas are low-grade pilocystic astrocytomas that generally occur in childhood; they often are bilateral and associated with neurofibromatosis type 1. The optic nerve shows fusiform thickening and often enhances with gadolinium on T1-weighted (fat-saturated) images. The entire optic system should be examined to evaluate for intracranial extension of the tumor. T2-weighted sequences are best for this purpose (see Chapter 2, Fig. 29).

Optic nerve sheath meningiomas generally occur in adults and may also be associated with neurofibromatosis. The lesion causes fusiform thickening along the optic nerve. Gadolinium enhancement often results in a tram-track pattern, with enhancement of the thickened nerve sheath but without abnormal enhancement of the nerve itself (see Chapter 1, Fig. 6). This tram-track pattern is not specific for meningiomas, however. The characteristic calcifications of an optic sheath meningioma may be detected by a gradient-recalled echo technique but are better seen by CT.

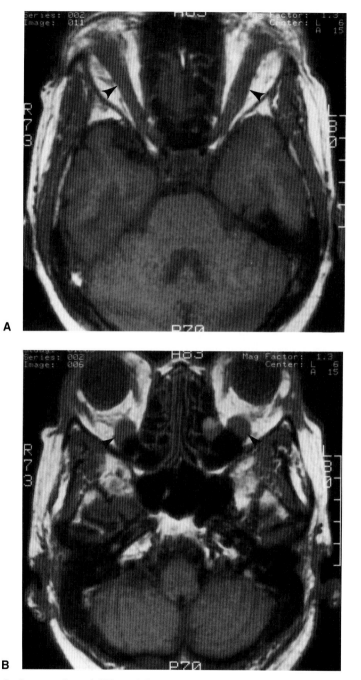

FIG. 8. Graves's disease. An axial T1-weighted image shows bilateral thickening of the (**A**) superior rectus muscles (*arrows*) and (**B**) inferior rectus muscles (*arrows*). Proptosis is also present.

Optic neuritis is usually caused by demyelination. Although variable, these lesions may produce a bright signal on T2-weighted sequences. In the acute phase, enhancement with gadolinium may occur. Sometimes, this enhancement has a tram-track pattern because of demyelination along the nerve periphery, and it can be confused with a meningioma.

NECK

Neck imaging in adults is best performed in a dedicated coil that has both an anterior and posterior component. Unlike a single anterior surface coil, this results is a near-homogeneous signal from similar tissues despite their anteroposterior position. A small child can be positioned in a head coil for even better neck imaging results. In most cases, coronal and axial T1- and axial T2-weighted FSE sequences are sufficient for diagnosis. For midline lesions, a sagittal sequence may also be useful. Tumors, inflammatory processes, and lymph nodes are all typically bright on T2-weighted images. Because the lymph node chains tend to be surrounded by fat in the neck, reducing or eliminating the fat signal (on T2-weighted sequences) with fat saturation is often helpful since this causes the regions of abnormality to be strikingly visible. T1-weighted images with contrast and fat saturation may also be useful.

Nasopharynx

The nasopharynx, the most cephalad aspect of the airway is important because of its intimate relationship with many critical structures of the upper neck, including the eustachian tubes and cranial nerves 3 to 6 and 9 to 12 (Fig. 9). It is separated by the fibrous pharyngobasilar fascia into superficial and deep compartments. The superficial compartment is called the mucosal space. It contains the muscles of deglutition (constrictor and palatal muscles), lymphoid tissue, and mucosa. The other relevant spaces to be discussed are in the deep compartment. The pharyngobasilar fascia acts as an anatomic barrier, limiting the spread of pathological processes between the superficial and deep compartmental structures.

The deep compartment is subdivided into multiple spaces. The parapharyngeal space is a triangular region containing mostly fat (bright on T1). It extends from the base of the skull to the hyoid bone, separating the muscles of mastication (masticator space, deep compartment), anterolaterally, from the muscles of deglutition (mucosal space, superficial compartment), anteromedially. The masticator space contains the muscles of mastication (pterygoids, masseter, and temporalis).

The carotid space borders the parapharyngeal space posteriorly. It contains the internal carotid artery, internal jugular vein, cranial nerves 9 to 12, and the cervical sympathetic plexus. The lateral retropharyngeal lymph nodes lie medial to the internal carotid artery and constitute the primary drainage for the nasopharynx. The parotid glands lie mainly lateral to the carotid sheath but do make contact with the parapharyngeal space (Fig. 9). Posterior to the nasopharynx, between the pharyngobasilar fossa and the prevertebral muscles (longus colli), lies the retropharyngeal space. This is a potential space that can act as a route of spread for tumors or infections.

Although the anatomy can seem overwhelming, the ability to develop a pertinent differential diagnosis often depends on the accurate localization of the pathologic process to one of the nasopharyngeal spaces. Fortunately, this can often be accomplished by assessing the related displacement of the adjacent fatty parapharyngeal space. Lateral displacement occurs with pathological conditions arising from the mucosal space (Table 7). Squamous cell carcinoma is the most common malignancy of the nasopharynx. It arises within the mucosal space, usually from within the fossa of Rosenmüller (Fig. 10.) Tumors typically spread along fascial planes, neural pathways, and lymphatic channels.

Medial displacement of the parapharyngeal space occurs with masses that arise from the masticator space or, sometimes, from the parotid gland (Table 8 and Fig. 11). Anterior

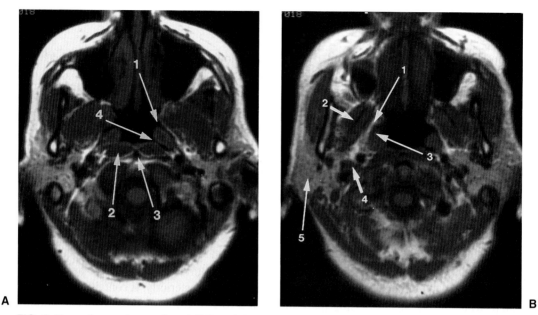

FIG. 9. Normal nasopharynx in axial T1-weighted images. **A:** Upper nasopharynx demonstrates eustachian tube orifices (*1*). The longus colli muscles (*2*) are posterior to the retropharyngeal space (*3*). The fossa of Rosenmüller is also seen (*4*). **B:** Lower nasopharynx demonstrates the triangular fatty (hyperintense) parapharyngeal space (*1*), which separates the muscles of mastication (masticator space, *2*) from the muscles of deglutition (mucosal space, *3*). The carotid space (*4*) and the parotid gland (*5*) border the parapharyngeal space posteriorly.

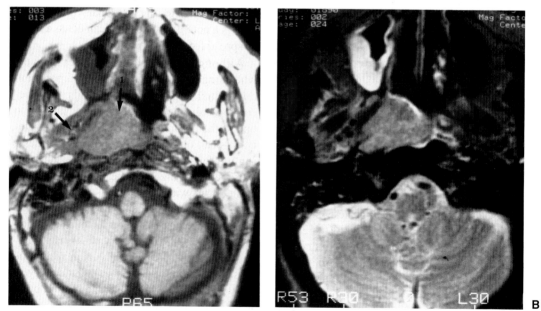

FIG. 10. Nasopharyngeal carcinoma (squamous cell). **A:** A T1-weighted axial image demonstrates an intermediate signal mass (*1*) within the mucosal space on the right, deviating the parapharyngeal space laterally (*2*). The mass occludes or obliterates the right eustachian tube, causing the patient to present with otitis media. **B:** A T2-weighted image shows the mass becoming hyperintense to adjacent tissues.

TABLE 7. *Differential diagnosis of medial mass, pushing parapharyngeal space laterally*

Nasopharyngeal carcinoma
Lymphoma
Minor salivary gland tumor

TABLE 8. *Differential diagnosis of lateral mass, pushing parapharyngeal space medially*

Dental abscess (masticator space)
Parotid tumor
Masticator space neoplasm (rare)
Neurofibroma

displacement occurs with pathological conditions in or around the carotid space (Table 9).

Oropharynx

The oropharynx is separated from the nasopharynx by the soft palate. Whether arising from the pharyngeal wall, base of tongue, tonsils, or palate, 90% of malignant lesions of the oropharynx are squamous cell carcinoma. The spread of disease is submucosal, along deep fascial planes, and into local lymph nodes. The nodal drainage is into the superior internal jugular chains and into the jugulodiagrastic nodes. Like most tumors, squamous cell carcinoma is nearly isointense to muscle on T1-weighted and hyperintense on T2-weighted sequences (Fig. 12). Benign masses of the oropharynx include hemangiomas (children), ectopic (lingual) thyroid, neurofibromas, and salivary tumors.

Larynx

The larynx extends from the epiglottis superiorly to the cricoid cartilage inferiorly. Except for the epiglottis, which performs both respiratory and digestive tract functions, the larynx is a respiratory organ. It is anatomically divided into three compartments: supra-

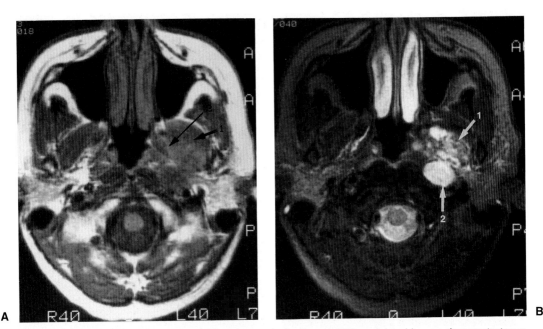

FIG. 11. Parotid mass (mixed-cell salivary tumor). **A:** An axial T1-weighted image demonstrates a mass (*1*), which is isointense with muscle, centered in the masticular space, pushing the parapharyngeal space (*2*) medially. **B:** A T2-weighted image demonstrates the heterogeneously, hyperintense mass (*1*) and a hyperintense, enlarged lateral pharyngeal lymph node (*2*).

TABLE 9. *Differential diagnosis of posterior mass, pushing parapharyngeal space anteriorly*

Adenopathy
Paraganglioma (chemodectoma)
Schwannoma
Abscess
Meningioma (rare)

glottic, glottic, and subglottic (Fig. 13). The supraglottic compartment contains the structures above the true cords to the epiglottis, whereas the compartment extending below the true cords to the cricoid cartilage is subglottic. The glottis is the level of the true vocal cords. These anatomic divisions are important because they are related to patterns of lymph node drainage, types of surgical procedures necessary for tumor resection, and prognosis.

Virtually all primary laryngeal malignancies are squamous cell carcinomas. They most commonly occur in the glottis (Fig. 14). Glottic tumors are often diagnosed early, while they are still confined to a vocal cord, because the pa-

tient develops hoarseness. The prognosis in these patients is excellent. If untreated, these tumors tend to spread to the anterior commissure where they can become bilateral and extend to the supra- or subglottic compartments and into the lymph nodes. The lymphatic drainage of the glottic and supraglottic compartments is into the superior internal jugular lymph node chain and the jugulodigastric nodes.

The prognosis of primary supraglottic or subglottic tumors is generally worse than that of glottic tumors because these lesions typically remain asymptomatic until they are large. Lymphatic drainage of the subglottic compartment is into the inferior internal jugular chain. The important features to note when evaluating laryngeal tumors are the following: (1) the presence of contralateral involvement, vertical extension (i.e., associated supraglottic, glottic, or subglottic spread), (2) adenopathy, and (3) involvement of the major vascular structures, especially the internal carotid arteries.

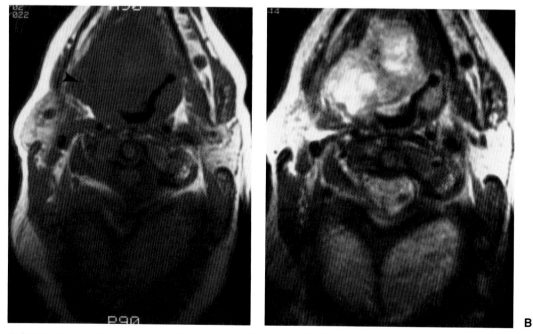

A   **B**

FIG. 12. Base of the tongue mass (squamous cell carcinoma). **A:** An axial T1-weighted image demonstrates a large mass at the tongue base on the right (*arrow*), which is isointense with muscle. **B:** A T2-weighted image demonstrates an increased signal intensity in the mass. The airway is narrowed.

Thyroid and Parathyroid Glands

In general, ultrasonography and scintigraphy are preferred over MRI for the evaluation of the thyroid gland. Scintigraphy can evaluate thyroid function. Ultrasonography can differentiate cystic from solid lesions better. Using MRI, most thyroid lesions are low or isointense in signal with the normal thyroid on T1 and hyperintense on T2 (Fig. 15). Malignant lesions cannot be differentiated from benign ones; MRI may be useful in selected patients to identify ectopic (substernal) thyroid tissue and define deep invasion of thyroid malignancies. It has also been used in differentiating recurrent thyroid cancer (bright on T2) from postoperative fibrosis (dark on T2).

Parathyroid adenomas are a relatively common cause of hypercalcemia. The sensitivity of MRI in detecting abnormal parathyroid glands is greater than that of ultrasonography, CT, or scintigraphy, especially in the preoperative localization of parathyroid adenomas. There are usually four parathyroid glands, two posterior to the upper poles of the thyroid and two posterior to the inferolateral aspects of the thyroid gland. The inferior glands are occasionally ectopic and may be located anywhere from the level of the jaw to the superior mediastinum. Normal parathyroid glands are often too small to visualize by imaging studies. Glands containing an adenoma are enlarged and generally identifiable. The signal characteristics may be variable, depending on the presence of hemorrhage or fibrosis, but they are usually isointense with the thyroid on T1-weighted and hyperintense on T2-weighted sequences (Fig. 15), making them conspicuous. Because lymph nodes and parathyroid adenomas have similar signal characteristics, a node may simulate an adenoma. The typical almond shape and medial location of a parathyroid adenoma can help in its differentiation from a node, which typically is rounded and laterally placed near the carotid sheath.

Brachial Plexus

The brachial plexus arises from the ventral nerve roots of C-5 to T-1. After the roots exit the spinal canal through their respective foramina, they course between the scalenus anterior and medius muscles, forming three trunks. These trunks then divide to form six divisions, which traverse the supraclavicular fossa, superior to the subclavian artery, entering the axilla. In the axilla, the six divisions surround the axillary artery to form three cords. The brachial plexus can generally be visualized in the neck, supraclavicular fossa, and axilla on MRI. Actual trunks, divisions, and cords also are sometimes resolved. The plexus in the neck and supraclavicular fossa are best seen on coronal and axial images, whereas the axillary portion is best seen sagittally (Fig. 16).

Under normal circumstances, the brachial plexus is surrounded by fat and is low in signal intensity on both T1- and T2-weighted images. Abnormalities intrinsic to the plexus include inflammatory processes or neurogenic tumors, such as schwannomas and neurofibromas (Fig. 17). Typically these abnormalities cause increased signal intensity within the plexus on T2-weighted images. In addition, neoplasms cause a mass-like expansion.

Probably the most common cause of symptoms referable to the brachial plexus is from extrinsic compression. This may occur in the presence of cervical ribs or bony abnormalities, sometimes causing thoracic outlet syndrome, or may occur in the presence of adjacent metastatic tumor (especially, lung and breast). The multiplanar abilities of MRI make it the procedure of choice for the evaluation of the brachial plexus. Sagittal images provide an accurate depiction of the plexus throughout its course.

Congenital Neck Abnormalities

The embryonic development of the brachial apparatus occurs from the 4th to 7th week of gestation. With further differentiation into structures of the head and neck, the brachial apparatus is obliterated. A brachial sinus, fistula, or cyst forms in the presence of residual brachial cell rests when incomplete obliteration occurs.

The location of the sinus, fistula, or cyst determines the level of origin from the brachial

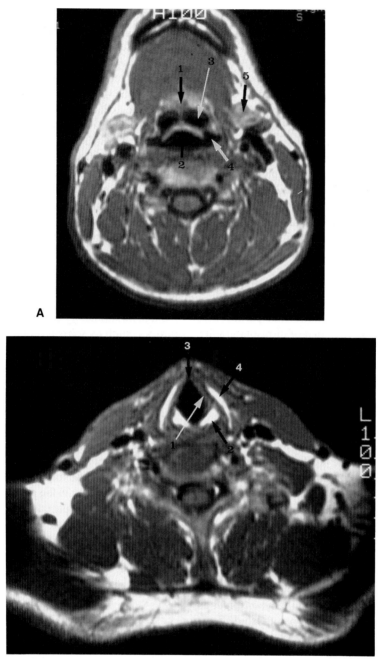

FIG. 13. Normal larynx in T1-weighted images. **A:** Supraglottal compartment at the level of the hyoid bone (*1*) demonstrates the epiglottis (*2*), valleculae (*3*), pyriform sinuses (*4*), and submandibular glands (*5*). **B:** Glottic compartment demonstrates the true vocal cords (*1*) attached to the arytenoid cartilage posteriorly (*2*) and the anterior commissure anteriorly (*3*). The thyroid cartilage is also seen (*4*).

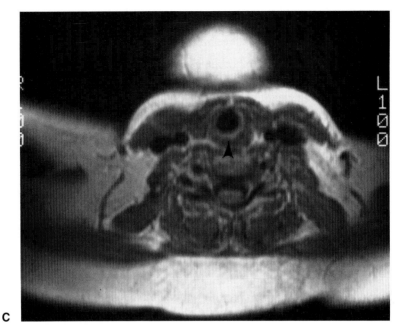

FIG. 13. *(continued)* **C:** Infraglottic compartment demonstrates the airway surrounded by the cricoid cartilage *(arrow)*.

apparatus. The second brachial apparatus is the level from which the majority of anomalies arise. Second brachial abnormalities can occur anywhere along a tract from the anterior junction of the middle and lower third of the sternocleidomastoid muscle, running deep to the platysma, ascending along the carotid sheath, passing between the internal and external carotid arteries, and ending cephalad near the tonsillar fossa. Most often however, the cyst lies along the carotid sheath (Fig. 18). Typically, brachial cleft cysts are fluid filled, with low T1- and high T2-weighted signals. The T1 signal may vary, however, depending on the protein content of the fluid.

Midline cysts are not of brachial origin but often arise from the thyroglossal duct. This duct is created during the embryonic descent of the thyroid gland from its origin at the foramen cecum to its resting position anterior to the trachea. Subsequent failure of complete obliteration of the thyroglossal duct can result in a cyst anywhere along its course. However,

most thyroglossal cysts are located near the hyoid bone (Fig. 19).

Hemangiomas of the head and neck are relatively common in children. They may be deeply invasive and disfiguring. Typically, MRI demonstrates an infiltrative mass that has a low signal intensity on T1-weighted and a high signal intensity on T2-weighted images (Fig. 20). T2-weighted fat-saturated images can be helpful in evaluating the extent of tissue invasion.

A cystic hygroma (lymphangioma) is an abnormality of the lymphatic system, usually involving the lower third of the neck, positioned in the posterior triangle. Cystic, painless, multiloculated, fluid-filled cavities form, probably as a result of abnormal connections to the main lymphatic channels. Typically, MRI demonstrates a thin-walled cystic mass, often with septations. The signal characteristics are typically those of water, i.e., a low signal intensity on T1 (unless hemorrhagic or infected) and a high signal intensity on T2-weighted sequences (Fig. 21).

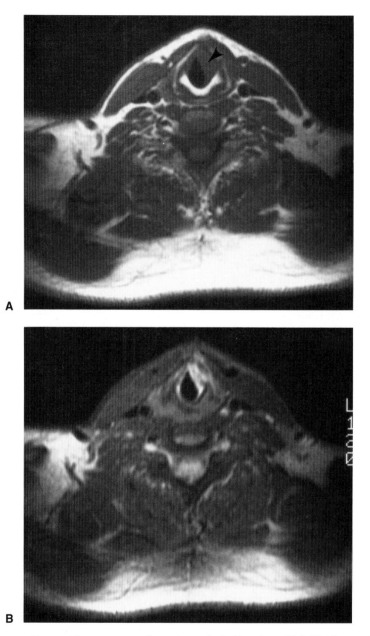

FIG. 14. Laryngeal tumors (squamous cell carcinoma). **A:** Vocal cord (glottic) tumor. A T1-weighted axial image demonstrates thickening of the left vocal cord (*arrow*). **B:** A T2-weighted image demonstrates the lesion's hyperintensity. The patient presented clinically with hoarseness.

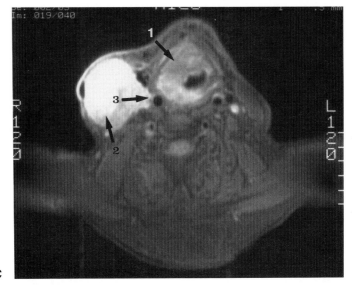

FIG. 14. *(continued)* **C:** Supraglottic tumor. A T2-weighted axial image shows a large hyperintense mass at the level of the false cords (*1*) associated with lymphadenopathy (*2*) in the superior internal jugular chain. The tumor crosses the midline to become nearly circumferential around the airway and, likely, invades the right internal carotid artery (*3*).

BIBLIOGRAPHY

Books

1. Som PM, Bergerson RT. *Head and neck imaging.* 2nd ed. St. Louis: Mosby Year Book;1991.
2. Higgins CB, Hricak H, Helms CA. *Magnetic resonance imaging of the body.* 2nd ed. New York: Raven Press;1992.

Journals

1. Tien RD, Chu PK, Hesselink JR, Szumoski J. Intra and paraorbital lesions: value of fat-suppression MR imaging with paramagnetic contrast enhancement. *AJNR Am J Neuroradiol* 1991;12:245–253.
2. MacFee MF, Putterman A, Valvassori GE, Campos M, Capek V. Orbital space-occupying lesions: role of computed tomography and magnetic resonance imaging. An analysis of 145 cases. *Radiol Clin North Am* 1987;25:529–559.
3. Sobel DF, Kelly W, Kjos BO, Char D, Brandt-Zawadski M, Norman D. MR imaging of orbital and ocular disease. *AJNR Am J Neuroradiol* 1985;6:259–264.
4. Mihara F, Gupta KL, Muryama S, Lee N, Bond JB, Haik BG. MR imaging of malignant uveal melanoma: role of pulse sequence and contrast agent. *AJR Am J Roentgenol* 1991;157:1087–1092.
5. Peyster RG, Shapir MD, Haik BG. Orbital metastasis: role of magnetic resonance imaging and computed tomography. *Radiol Clin North Am* 1987;25:647–662.
6. Hopper KD, Sherman JL, Boal DKB, Eggle KKD. CT and MR imaging of the pediatric orbit. *Radiographics* 1992;12:485–503.
7. Bilanuik LT, Atlas SW, Zimmerman RA. Magnetic resonance imaging of the orbit. *Radiol Clin North Am* 1987;25:509–528.
8. Flanders AE, Espinosa GA, Markiewitz DA, Howell DD. Orbital lymphoma: role of CT and MRI. *Radiol Clin North Am* 1987;25:601–613.
9. Hosten N, Sander B, Cordes M, Schubert CJ, Shorner W, Felix R. Graves ophthalmopathy: MR imaging of the orbits. *Radiology* 1989;172:759–762.
10. Hendrix LE, Kneeland JE, Haughton VM, et al. MR imaging of optic nerve lesions: value of gadopentetate dimegumine and fat-suppression technique. *AJR Am J Roentgenol* 1990;155:849–854.
11. Harnesburger HR, Osborn AG. Differential diagnosis of head and neck lesions based on their space of origin. The suprahyoid part of the neck. *AJR Am J Roentgenol* 1991;157:147–154.
12. Teresi LM, Lufkin RB, Vinuela F, Dietrich RB, Wilson GH, Bentson JR, Hanafee WN. MR imaging of the nasopharynx and floor of the middle cranial fossa. Part 1. Normal anatomy. *Radiology* 1987;164:811–816.
13. Teresi LM, Lufkin RB, Vinuela F, Dietrich RB, Wilson GH, Bentson JR, Hanafee WN. MR imaging of the nasopharynx and floor of the middle cranial fossa. Part II. Malignant Tumors. *Radiology* 1987;164:817–821.
14. Som PM, Sacher M, Stollman AL, Biller HF, Lawson W. Common tumors of the parapharyngeal space: refined imaging diagnosis. *Radiology* 1988;169:81–85.
15. Kassel EE, Keller MA, Kucharczyk W. MRI of the floor of the mouth, tongue and oropharynx. *Radiol Clin North Am* 1989;27:331–351.

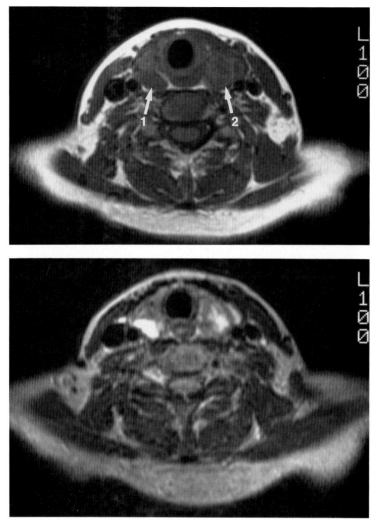

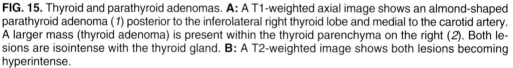

FIG. 15. Thyroid and parathyroid adenomas. **A:** A T1-weighted axial image shows an almond-shaped parathyroid adenoma (*1*) posterior to the inferolateral right thyroid lobe and medial to the carotid artery. A larger mass (thyroid adenoma) is present within the thyroid parenchyma on the right (*2*). Both lesions are isointense with the thyroid gland. **B:** A T2-weighted image shows both lesions becoming hyperintense.

16. Teresi LM, Lufkin RB, Hanafee WN. Magnetic resonance imaging of the larynx. *Radiol Clin North Am* 1989;27:393–406.
17. Curtin HD. Imaging of the larynx: current concepts. *Radiology* 1989;173:1–11.
18. Kier R, Herfkens RJ, Blinder RA, Leight GS, Utz JA, Silverman PM. MRI with surface coils for parathyroid tumors: preliminary investigation. *AJR* 1986; 147:497–500.
19. Aufferman W, Guis M, Tavares NJ, Clark OH, Higgins CB. MR signal intensity of parathyroid adenomas: correlation with histopathology. *AJR Am J Roentgenol* 1989;153:873–876.
20. Blair DN, Rapoport S, Sostman HD, Blair OC. Normal brachial plexus: MR imaging. *Radiology* 1987; 165:763–767.
21. Castagno AA, Shuman WP. MR imaging in clinically suspected brachial plexus tumor. *AJR Am J Roentgenol* 1987;149:1219–1222.
22. Rapoport S, Blair DN, McCarthy SM, Desser TS, Hammers LW, Sostman HD. Brachial plexus: correlation of MR imaging with CT and pathologic findings. *Radiology* 1988;167:161–165.
23. Benson MT, Dalen K, Mancuso AA, Kerr HH, Cacciarelli AA, MacFee MF. Congenital anomalies of the brachial apparatus: embryology and pathologic anatomy. *Radiographics* 1992;12:943–960.
24. Reede DL, Bergeron RT, Som PM. CT of the thyroglossal duct cysts. *Radiology* 1985;157:121–125.
25. Itoh K, Nishimura K, Togashi K, Fujisawa I, Nakano Y, Itoh H, Torizuka K. MR imaging of a cavernous hemangioma of the face and neck. *J Comput Assist Tomogr* 1986;10:831–835.
26. Zadvinskis DP, Benson MT, Kerr HH, et al. Congenital malformations of the cervicothoracic lymphatic system: embryology and pathogenesis. *Radiographics* 1992;12:1175–1189.

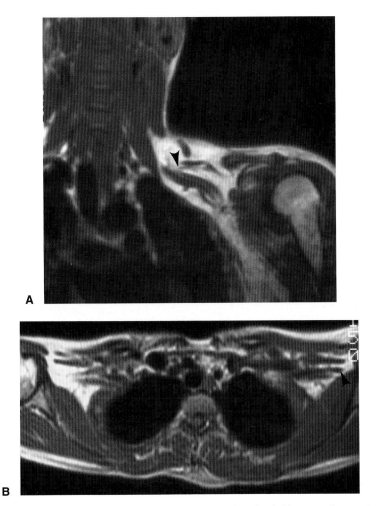

FIG. 16. Normal brachial plexus. **A,B:** T1-weighted coronal and axial images demonstrate the supraclavicular portion of the low-signal-intensity brachial plexus (*arrows*) surrounded by high-signal-intensity fat.

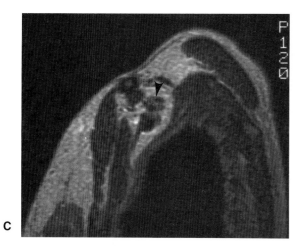

C

FIG. 16. *(continued)* **C:** A T2-weighted sagittal image demonstrates the axillary portion of the plexus (*arrow*), which remains low in signal intensity.

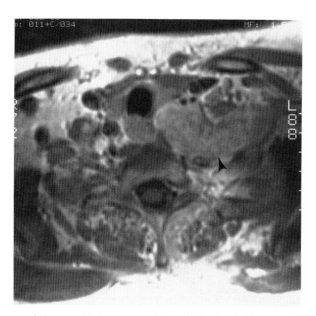

FIG. 17. Neurofibroma of the brachial plexus. A T1-weighted axial image with gadolinium shows a mildly enhancing mass (*arrow*) within the left brachial plexus.

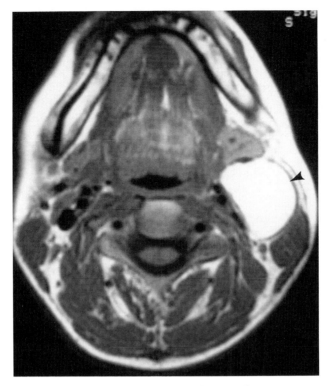

FIG. 18. Second brachial cleft cyst. An axial T1-weighted image demonstrates a well-circumscribed homogeneous mass (*arrow*) that lies adjacent to the carotid sheath on the left. The hyperintense signal is caused by proteinaceous fluid. (Courtesy of Jerome Barakos, MD. California Pacific Medical Center.)

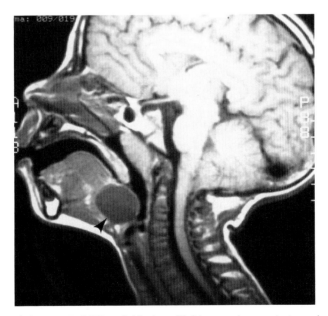

FIG. 19. Thyroglossal duct cyst. A T1-weighted sagittal image demonstrates a low-signal-intensity cyst (*arrow*) in the midline neck at the level of the hyoid bone.

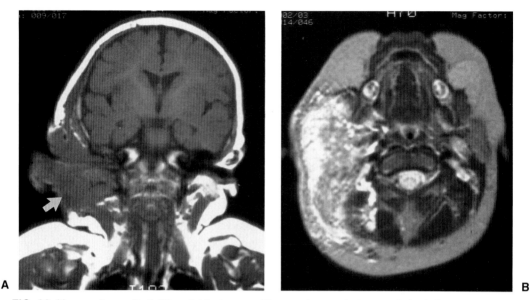

FIG. 20. Hemangioma. **A:** A T1-weighted coronal image demonstrates a relatively low signal mass (*arrow*) arising from the right neck. It obliterates the right external auditory canal and expands the auricle. **B:** A T2-weighted axial image shows hyperintense signal and the invasive character of the mass.

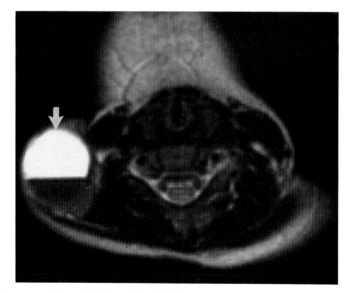

FIG. 21. Cystic hygroma. An axial T2-weighted FSE image demonstrates a well-defined cystic mass in the right neck (*arrow*). The fluid–fluid level is caused by hemorrhage within the cyst.

5

Chest

INTRODUCTION

Magnetic resonance imaging (MRI) of the chest is probably the most challenging of any body region because of the unavoidable motion of the lungs, heart, and rapidly flowing blood. To obtain a diagnostic image, careful attention must be paid to the imaging parameters. Respiratory compensation and cardiac gating are essential.

The respiratory compensation belt is an accordion-like tube. For best results, it should be wrapped around the chest or abdomen in the general region being scanned. It should be pulled snug enough such that expansion of the belt occurs with inspiration. Instructions should be given to the patient to take regular medium-sized breaths during the scans, avoiding deep breaths or sighs.

Cardiac gating can be performed by the use of electrocardiographic (ECG) leads or by a peripheral lead on the patient's finger or toe. In general, for chest imaging ECG tracing gives a sharper, better defined R wave than does peripheral gating. This allows image acquisition to initiate more precisely at the same point in the cardiac cycle each time, reducing image blurring and artifacts.

The ECG leads should be placed on the patient's left back (right for dextrocardia) near the level of the scapula. This allows the leads to remain motionless with respiration in the supine position. In the magnetic field, blood flow induces a current that superimposes on the ECG. This artifact may make ECG interpretation difficult and induce artifactual triggers. The posterior placement of leads will also tend to minimize these artifacts. When placed anteriorly, the leads (wires) move within a magnetic field during respiration, generating a voltage between them that can interfere with detection of the patient's intrinsic cardiac depolarization.

Experience varies on the optimal lead placement pattern for the posterior chest. An easy pattern that reliably produces a signal of adequate magnitude for gating is a square pattern. The "arm" leads are positioned at the same vertical height, near the upper scapula, one paraspinous to the left and the second near the posterior axially line. At the same vertical height near the inferior aspect of the scapula, the "leg" leads are placed. The "left leg" can be placed in the inferior axilla.

For most applications in the chest, a diagnostic study can be obtained by acquiring cardiac-gated T1 coronal and T1- and T2-weighted axial sequences. For cardiac studies, if the anatomy is the major concern, the T2-weighted sequence can be eliminated, but virtually all cardiac studies benefit from the addition of a cine sequence, usually in the axial plane.

MEDIASTINUM (NONCARDIAC)

The mediastinum is divided into three compartments: anterior, middle, and posterior. The anterior mediastinum is the space between the sternum and the anterior pericardium, aorta, and brachiocephalic vessels. The major organ occupying this space is the thymus gland. The middle mediastinum contains the pericardium, heart, great vessels, trachea, and main stem bronchi. Between the posterior pericardium and the spinal column is the posterior mediastinum. Major structures contained in this space are the descending aorta, esophagus, sympathetic nerve trunks, and peripheral nerves as they exit the neural foramina of the spine.

Localizing pathological conditions into a mediastinal compartment helps to formulate a differential diagnosis for mediastinal masses because primary tumors arise from the anatomical structures contained in that compartment. Common to all compartments, however, are lymph nodes. Adenopathy may represent primary disease (lymphoma) or metastatic spread of tumor, or it may be related to inflammatory processes.

Similar to computed tomography (CT), MRI uses size criteria to determine whether lymph nodes are likely to be normal or abnormal. MRI has not been able to distinguish benign from malignant nodes reliably by the signal characteristics. In general, similar to lymph nodes elsewhere in the body, mediastinal and hilar nodes are considered abnormal by size criteria when they are 1 cm or larger. The search for adenopathy should include inspection of the internal mammary chains, perivascular space (around the great vessels), aortopulmonary window, right paratracheal space, pre- and subcarinal spaces, azygoesophageal recess, paraspinous spaces, and lung hila. Coronal images may be helpful. Typically, the nodes are best seen on the T1-weighted images because they are low in signal intensity, surrounded by high-signal-intensity fat, with the blood vessels black. The adenopathy is then confirmed on a T2-weighted sequence, in which it is typically hyperintense to fat (Fig. 1). Unlike with CT, intravenous contrast is seldom needed in evaluation of adenopathy by MRI.

In addition to adenopathy, the differential diagnosis for a mass in the anterior mediastinum includes thymoma, germ cell tumor, and thyroid tissue. The normal thymus gland in a young child fills the anterior mediastinum, is quadrilateral in shape, and has convex contours (Fig. 2). It may extend to the retrocaval space. After age 5 years, the thymus takes on a more triangular appearance, becoming bilobed and oval and involuting during adulthood. The thymus is mildly hyperintense to muscle on T1-weighted and increases in signal on T2-weighted sequences, appearing similar to that of fat on T2-weighted images. This occasionally presents a problem when evaluating the patient for adenopathy, especially in children, because the thymus has signal characteristics similar to a nodal mass. The patient's age, the expected shape of the normal thymus gland, and the presence or absence of adenopathy elsewhere in the mediastinum should be taken into consideration when evaluating for lymphadenopathy in the anterior mediastinum.

Thymomas occur in adults and may be associated with myasthenia gravis. They are malignant in 30% of cases. The gland is typically enlarged, and unlike thymic hyperplasia, it loses its normal bilobed, oval contour. Its signal characteristics are similar to the normal gland, but more internal heterogeneity and septations are generally present. Local invasion of fat, vessels, or pericardium may be seen with malignant thymomas.

Germ cell tumors arise from embryonic cell rests in the anterior mediastinum. They may be benign or malignant. The most common malignant tumor is a teratoma. It can often be differentiated from a thymoma and from adenopathy by the presence of fat (confirmed by a fat-saturated sequence) and calcification, which is dark on all sequences and blooms on gradient-recalled echo (GRE) imaging. These lesions are heterogeneous is appearance. A retrosternal goiter is generally well circumscribed and isointense to the thyroid gland on both T1- and T2-weighted sequences. Usually a connection to a thyroid lobe within the neck can be demonstrated (Fig. 3).

Major noncardiovascular considerations for masses occupying the middle mediastinum include adenopathy and abnormalities arising from the tracheobronchial tree. Bronchogenic cysts, duplication cysts, and pericardial cysts are well visualized with MRI. They are well circumscribed and high in signal intensity on T2-weighted sequences. Their T1 signal is vari-

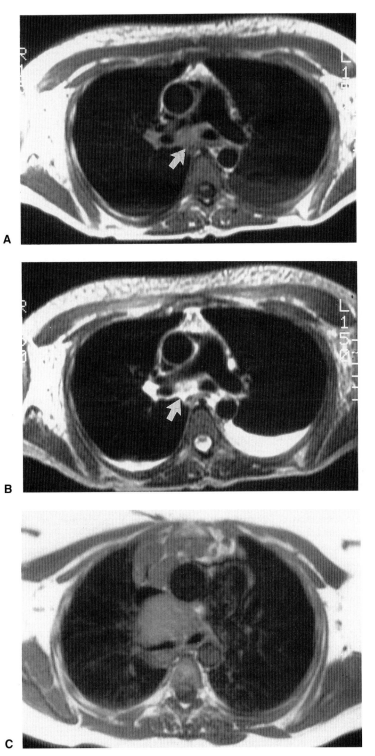

FIG. 1. A: Adenopathy (lymphoma). A T1-weighted cardiac-gated axial image shows low-signal-intensity lymph nodes in the subcarinal region (*arrow*) and within the right hilum. **B:** A T2-weighted cardiac-gated image demonstrates the nodes to be hyperintense. **C:** A T1-weighted axial cardiac-gated image demonstrates an example of massive adenopathy.

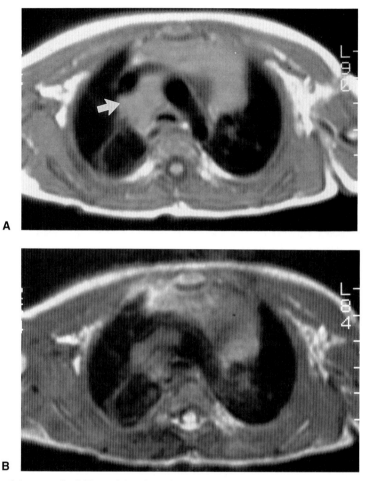

FIG. 2. Normal thymus. **A:** A T1-weighted cardiac-gated axial image demonstrates the quadrilateral shape of the thymus, with thymic tissue extending into the retrocaval position (*arrow*). The gland is mildly hyperintense to muscle. **B:** A T2-weighted cardiac-gated sequence shows the thymus becoming increasingly hyperintense to muscle.

able, depending on the protein content and the presence of hemorrhage (Fig. 4.) Bronchogenic carcinoma, like most other neoplasms tend to be nearly isointense with muscle on T1-weighted and hyperintense on T2-weighted sequences. Particularly in relation to vascular structures, MRI can be useful in staging these tumors. Coronal images may be especially helpful in evaluating the lung apexes and the aortopulmonary window. T2-weighted images may help in assessing postobstructive atelectasis *versus* tumor. Except in selected cases these lesions are usually evaluated by CT, primarily because it allows superior assessment of associated lung abnormalities.

In addition to adenopathy, neurogenic tumors and esophageal abnormalities are the major differential diagnostic considerations for a posterior mediastinal mass. Whether arising from the sympathetic chains (ganglioneuroma or neuroblastoma) or from the peripheral nerves (neurofibroma or neurilemmoma), neurogenic masses are paraspinous in location and hyperintense on T2-weighted sequences (Fig. 5). Most are nearly isointense with muscle on T1. Axial images are useful to demonstrate intraspinal involvement through the neural foramina.

The normal esophagus is isointense with muscle on both T1- and T2-weighted se-

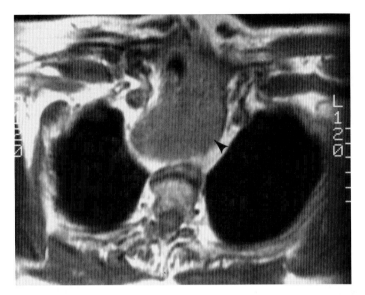

FIG. 3. Retrosternal goiter. An axial T1-weighted cardiac-gated image demonstrates a large retrosternal mass (*arrow*). It was continuous with the left thyroid in the neck.

quences. Because it is readily distensible and lacks a serosa (relative barrier for tumor spread), esophageal cancer tends to present late. By the time clinical symptoms occur, local invasion and metastatic tumor are present in many patients. Similar to other tumors, esophageal carcinoma is isointense with muscle on T1-weighted and hyperintense on T2-weighted sequences.

In general, CT and MRI are nearly equivalent in their accuracy in predicting the resectability of esophageal carcinoma (84% and 87%, respectively). Important considerations in resectability include the invasion of the trachea, bronchi, descending aorta, pericardium, and left atrium. To exclude local invasion, the multiplanar capability of MRI is useful in demonstrating an intact fat plane between the

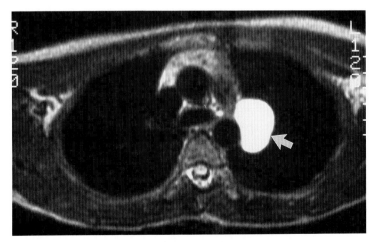

FIG. 4. Bronchogenic cyst. An axial T2-weighted cardiac-gated image demonstrates a homogeneously hyperintense mass in the middle mediastinum (*arrow*). It arose from the proximal left upper lobe bronchus.

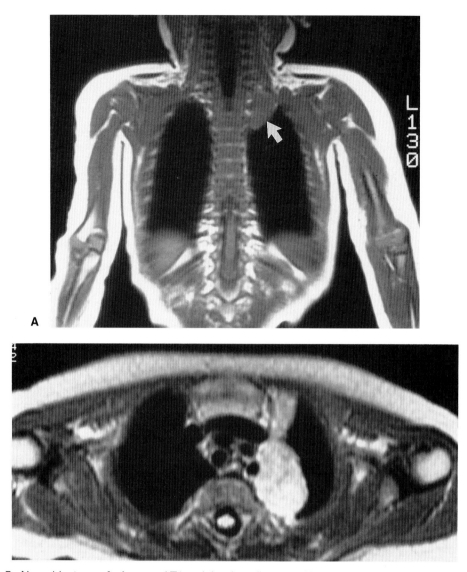

FIG. 5. Neuroblastoma. **A:** A coronal T1-weighted cardiac-gated image reveals an oval paraspinous mass (*arrow*), which is isointense to muscle. **B:** An axial T2-weighted cardiac-gated image. The mass becomes hyperintense and extends anteriorly, coming in contact with the great vessels (middle mediastinum).

tumor and the heart (best evaluated on T1-weighted sequence). This is less reliable for the aortic invasion, however. The fat plane between the normal esophagus and descending aorta is often effaced in the absence of pathological conditions. Reliance on a totally intact fat plane in this location can lead to increased false-positive diagnoses. Obliteration of the triangular fat space between the esophagus (at the site of the tumor), the descending aorta, and spine appears to be a reliable means of predicting tumor invasion of the aorta (Fig. 6).

Tracheal or bronchial invasion can be reliably predicted when the tumor can be seen extending to the lumen of the airway.

LUNGS

Pulmonary nodules, when present, are often detected on MRI. Primary and metastatic malignancies tend to be of low signal intensity on T1 and high signal intensity on T2 (Fig. 7). In general, however, CT is the preferred imaging modality for pulmonary evaluation. It offers greater spatial resolution, is not hampered by magnetic susceptibility artifact in the presence of air, and is less prone to motion artifacts than is MRI. Also, CT detects more small nodules than does MRI and is better able to evaluate lung segmental anatomy and interstitial and alveolar disease.

PERICARDIUM

The normal pericardium can be seen on MRI, outlined by fat along its internal and external surfaces. It measures 1 to 2 mm in thickness. A pericardial thickness of 3 to 4 mm or greater is abnormal and can be diagnostic for constrictive pericarditis in the proper clinical setting (Fig. 8). Visible pericardium around the entire heart also raises the suspicion of abnormal pericardium. With constrictive pericarditis, the pericardial thickening is often confined to the right side of the heart and associated with right atrial enlargement. The right ventricle is usually normal in size. This condition can be differentiated from restrictive cardiomyopathy, which might also present with right atrial enlargement, by its lack of pericardial thickening.

Pericardial effusions are low in signal intensity on both T1- and T2-weighted images (secondary to proton dephasing, which is produced by fluid sloshing during the cardiac activity). Because pericardial fluid is contained between the visceral and parietal layers of the pericardium, the low-signal-intensity fluid can mimic pericardial thickening. These two conditions can be differentiated on a cine sequence, however. With the GRE cine sequence, the sloshing pericardial effusion becomes bright (high signal intensity) whereas thickened pericardium remains dark (low signal intensity). Hemopericardium, unlike a simple pericardial effusion, may be bright (high signal) on T1-weighted sequences.

HEART

When evaluating the heart, either for congenital malformations or acquired disease, it is useful to have a systematic search pattern. One such pattern is to start in the superior and inferior vena cavae and follow the course of a hypothetical red blood cell. It should enter the right atrium, pass into the ventricle, proceed out the pulmonary arteries returning through the pulmonary veins to the left atrium, and then pass to the left ventricle and out the aorta. This ensures that the connections of the heart and vessels are correct. As each chamber or vessel is entered, the size of the chamber or vessel, its thickness, the signal of the myocardium, and the competency of the cardiac valves should be assessed. Septal defects should also be excluded. Although the atrial septum may seem to disappear on spin–echo cardiac-gated images near the fossa ovalis, cine MRI is helpful in evaluating possible defects.

Myocardial Infarction

Normal myocardium is low to intermediate in signal intensity on both T1- and T2-weighted, cardiac-gated images. The left ventricular anterior, inferior, lateral, and septal walls are fairly uniform in thickness. Some variation in wall thickness is expected on cardiac-gated images, however, depending on when in the cardiac cycle (systole or diastole) each image was acquired.

Because of the associated myocardial edema, an acute myocardial infarct becomes bright (high signal intensity) on T2-weighted images. With time, the edema resolves, and the myocardial wall becomes thin and low to intermediate in signal intensity on T2-weighted sequences. This represents scarring in chronic myocardial infarction. Gadolinium is also useful in delineating the presence of acute myocardial infarction because the abnormal region of myocardium enhances on delayed T1-weighted images (Fig. 9). Chronic infarction tends to be nonenhancing. Abnormal wall motion as a result of infarction can also be seen on a cardiac cine sequence, which displays the heart beating as if in real time. Normally, the left ventricular walls and septum should move vigorously and symmetrically in unison to contract the ventricular cavity during systole.

Cardiac Masses

Cardiac masses are well seen on MRI. Its diagnostic accuracy is better than echocardiog-

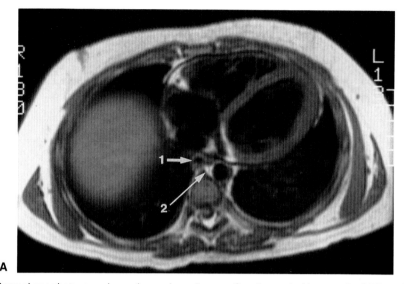

FIG. 6. Normal esophagus and esophageal carcinoma. Cardiac-gated image. **A:** A T1-weighted axial scan of the normal esophagus (*1*) demonstrates isointensity to muscle. A triangular fat-filled space (*2*) is present between the esophagus, descending aorta, and spine.

raphy and is generally used to define the size of a mass and its relationship to other cardiac and vascular structures. A common intracardiac mass is a thrombus (Fig. 10), which is usually found within the left atrium or left ventricle. A thrombus can be differentiated from primary and metastatic tumors on T1-weighted cardiac-gated images by the administration of gadolinium. Tumors generally enhance, whereas thrombi do not.

Cardiac Function and Valvular Disease

Cine MRI provides a multilevel tomographic view of the heart through the cardiac cycle. When each level is viewed as a movie (usually at sixteen frames per second), the beating heart can be evaluated. Because this is a GRE sequence, the myocardial walls are intermediate in signal intensity, and the flowing blood within the chambers is high in signal intensity (bright). This technique allows an assessment of wall motion, ventricular function, and chamber volumes.

Valvular disease can also be detected and its severity estimated using cine MRI. Valvular regurgitation is seen as a low-intensity (dark) jet extending from the affected valve into the otherwise hyperintense flowing blood. At the correct cardiac phase, it is seen in the cardiac chamber proximal to the valve. A similar low-intensity jet can be seen in valvular stenosis except that the low-intensity jet extends into the cardiac chamber or vessel distal to the valve. Regurgitation or stenotic jets are of low signal intensities because of their relative high velocity and inherent turbulence.

Congenital Heart Disease

In congenital heart disease, MRI provides a noninvasive technique for visualizing congenital malformations of the heart and associated vessels. The chamber size, vascular connections, septal defects, and luminal size of the associated aorta and pulmonary vessels can be determined. This information is important in preoperative planning and postsurgical

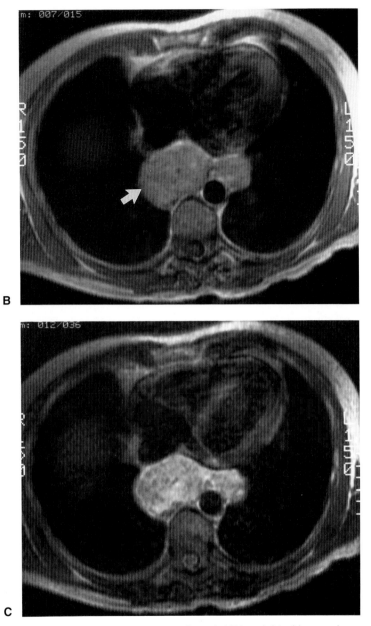

FIG. 6. *(continued)* **B:** Esophageal carcinoma. An axial T1-weighted image demonstrates a large posterior mediastinal mass (*arrow,* arising from the esophagus). The normal triangular fat space between the esophagus, aorta, and spine has been obliterated, suggesting invasion of the descending aorta. A thin hyperintense fat plane is present, which separates the mass from the heart, suggesting invasion of the pericardium and heart has not occurred. **C:** An axial T2-weighted image demonstrates increased hyperintensity of the mass.

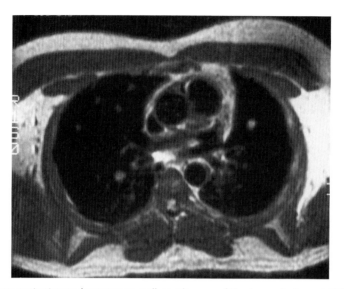

FIG. 7. Pulmonary metastases (squamous cell carcinoma of the larynx). An axial T2-weighted cardiac-gated image demonstrates multiple lung nodules.

assessment of cardiac status. Cardiac-gated T1-weighted images are indicated to demonstrate the cardiac anatomy, usually in the axial and, sometimes, coronal or sagittal projections. This should always be accompanied by a cine sequence (images usually in the axial projection). Often, anatomy that is confusing on the cardiac-gated T1-weighted images becomes clear when viewed as a movie with cine, which demonstrates blood flow through the cardiac cycle. T2-weighted images are rarely needed.

When evaluating congenital cardiac malformations, there is no substitute for experience and an understanding of developmental anatomy, but there are a few simple concepts that are often useful. These rules should be used carefully because they are not true in all cases. Increased systolic pressure within a cardiac chamber (e.g., with aortic stenosis) causes muscular hypertrophy without chamber dilatation (until late in the disease process). Increased blood volume through a chamber (e.g., through an atrial septal defect) causes chamber enlargement without muscular hypertrophy. It's important to know whether the patient is cyanotic or acyanotic. If acyanotic, a left-to-right shunt or a left-sided outflow obstruction is suspected. Shunt lesions include atrial septal de-

fect (which causes right-sided enlargement), ventricular septal defect or patent ductus arteriosus (both cause left-sided enlargement), and partial anomalous pulmonary venous connections.

In the presence of cyanosis, a right-to-left shunt is present. Disorders to consider are tetralogy of Fallot (Fig. 11) and transposition. Both have ventricular septal defects with pulmonic stenosis. The heart size tends to be normal. Tricuspid atresia (atrial septal defect), Ebstein's anomaly, hypoplastic left heart, truncus arteriosus, and total anomalous pulmonary venous return are also cyanotic lesions. They tend to have cardiac enlargement. A velocity-encoded sequence may be useful to evaluate shunt lesions. This is acquired much like a cine but also yields information related to blood flow direction and quantitative flow measurements, allowing shunt flow quantification.

THORACIC AORTA

Similar to congenital heart disease, MRI provides a noninvasive technique for evaluating congenital abnormalities of the aortic arch. Vascular rings resulting from a right aortic arch with an aberrant left subclavian artery are a rel-

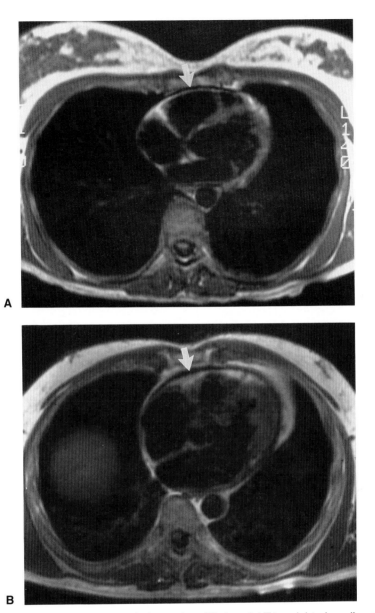

FIG. 8. Normal pericardium and constrictive pericarditis in axial T1-weighted cardiac-gated images. **A:** Thin, hypointense, normal pericardium (*arrow*) is shown, which is best seen along the anterior heart margin. It is outlined by hyperintense fat. **B:** Pericardial thickening (*arrow*) in a 45-year-old patient with constrictive pericarditis.

atively common abnormality requiring surgical repair (Fig. 12). Aortic coarctations can also be demonstrated (Fig. 13). An accurate diagnosis and demonstration of the associated vascular anatomy is important in preoperative assessment. The origins of the great vessels, the length of the coarctation, and the presence of collateral circulation can be determined.

Aortic dissection is an acquired abnormality resulting from blood dissecting into the media of the vessel. This results in an intimal flap, dividing the aorta into a true and false lumen. Aortic dissections are classified as two types. Type A involves the aorta proximal to the ligamentum arteriosum but may extend distally. It requires emergency surgical repair; the

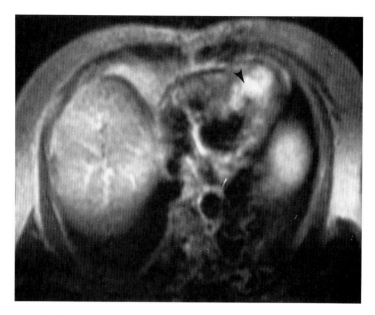

FIG. 9. Acute myocardial infarction. An axial T1-weighted cardiac-gated image with gadolinium demonstrates apical and septal enhancement (*arrow*), indicating an acute myocardial infarction.

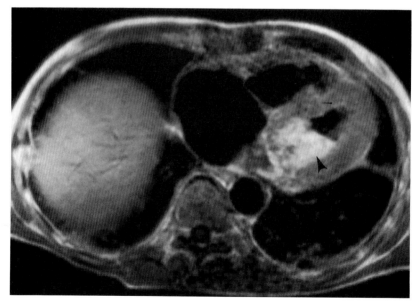

FIG. 10. Cardiac mass (thrombus). An axial T1-weighted cardiac-gated image demonstrates a hyperintense mass (*arrow*) within the left ventricle.

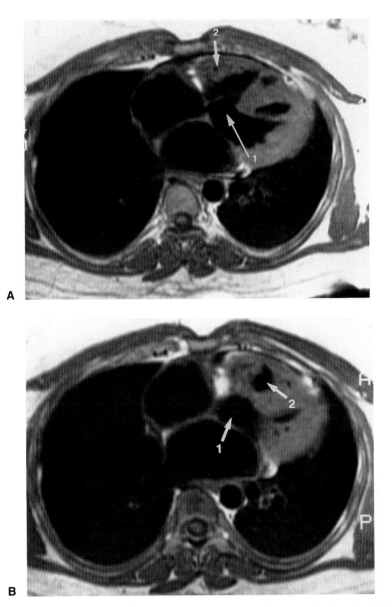

FIG. 11. Tetralogy of Fallot in axial T1-weighted cardiac-gated images. **A:** A large perimembranous ventricular septal defect (*1*) is present with right ventricular hypertrophy (*2*). **B:** The aorta overrides the ventricular septal defect (*1*). Infundibular pulmonic stenosis is also present (*2*).

mortality rate is 1% per hour on the first day. Type B dissections involve only the aorta distal to the ligamentum arteriosum and are often managed medically (blood pressure reduction). Rupture of either type A or B is a surgical emergency and is seen as an abnormal soft tissue signal (blood) in the mediastinum.

Cardiac-gated axial T1-weighted and GRE images are superior alternatives to contrast-enhanced CT for the evaluation of a suspected aortic dissection (Fig. 14). Imaging should begin just cephalad to the aortic arch and extend below the level of the ligamentum arteriosum. If a dissection is encountered, scanning

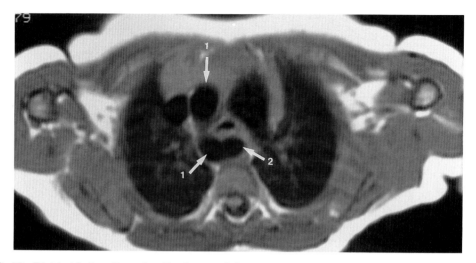

FIG. 12. Right-sided aortic arch with aberrant left subclavian artery. A T1-weighted axial cardiac-gated image shows a right-sided ascending and descending aorta (*1*). The origin of the aberrant left subclavian is seen within a characteristic diverticulum (*2*).

should continue to its caudal aspect (often into the abdomen). To diagnose a dissection, an intimal flap must be visualized. The T1-weighted sequence shows the anatomy best. A GRE sequence is helpful in demonstrating flow within the dissection and associated aortic branches. Velocity-encoded images may provide the most sensitive and specific tool. The axial plane is preferred for diagnosis. Although sometimes used, the left anterior oblique plane can be difficult to interpret.

BIBLIOGRAPHY

Books

1. Higgins CB, Hricak H, Helms CA. *Magnetic resonance imaging of the body.* 2nd ed. New York: Raven Press; 1992.

Journals

1. Lanzer P, Botvinick EH, Schiller NB, et al. Cardiac imaging using gated magnetic resonance. *Radiology* 1984;150:121–127.
2. Dimick RN, Hedlund LW, Herfkens RJ, Fram EK, Utz J. Optimizing electrocardiograph electrode placement for cardiac-gated magnetic resonance imaging. *Invest Radiol* 1987;22:17–22.
3. Siegel MJ, Glazer HS, Wiener JL, Molina PL. Normal and abnormal thymus in childhood: MR imaging. *Radiology* 1989;172:367–371.
4. Templeton PA, Caskey CI, Zerhouni EA. Current uses of CT and MR imaging in the staging of lung cancer. *Radiol Clin North Am* 1990;28:631–646.
5. Webb WR, Gatsonis C, Zerhouni EA, Heelan RT, Glazer GM, Francis IR, McNeil BJ. CT and MR imaging in staging non-small cell bronchogenic carcinoma: report of the radiologic diagnostic oncology group. *Radiology* 1991;178:705–713.
6. Takashima S, Takeuchi N, Shiozaki H, et al. Carcinoma of the esophagus: CT vs. MR imaging in determining resectability. *AJR Am J Roentgenol* 1911; 156:297–302.

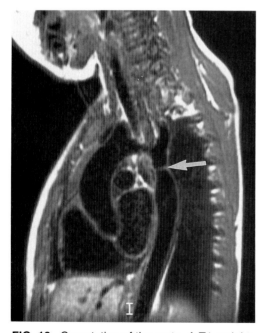

FIG. 13. Coarctation of the aorta. A T1-weighted sagittal cardiac-gated image shows focal aortic narrowing (*arrow*) at the level of the ligamentum arteriosum.

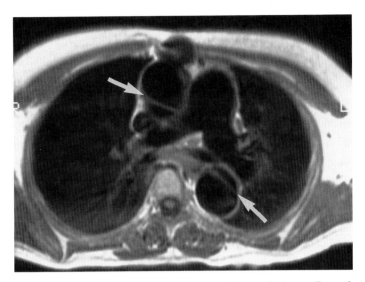

FIG. 14. Aortic dissection. A T1-weighted axial sequence demonstrates a dissection within the ascending and descending aorta. The intimal flap (*arrows*) separates the true lumen from the false lumen.

7. Muller NL, Gamsu G, Webb WR. Pulmonary nodules: detection using magnetic resonance and computed tomography. *Radiology* 1985;155:687–690.

8. Sechtem U, Tscholakoff D, Higgins CB. MRI of the normal pericardium. *AJR Am J Roentgenol* 1986; 147:239–244.

9. Sechtem U, Tscholakoff D, Higgins CB. MRI of the abnormal pericardium. *AJR Am J Roentgenol* 1986;147:245–252.

10. Fisher MR, McNamara MT, Higgins CB. Acute myocardial infarction: MR evaluation in 29 patients. *AJR Am J Roentgenol* 1987;148:247–251.

11. vanDijkman PR, van der Wall EE, de Roos A, et al. Acute, subacute, and chronic myocardial infarction: quantitative analysis of gadolinium-enhanced MR images. *Radiology* 1991;180:147–151.

12. Sechtem U, Pflufelder PW, White RD, Gould RG, Holt W, Lipton MJ, Higgins CB. Cine MR imaging: potential for the evaluation of cardiovascular function. *AJR Am J Roentgenol* 1987;148:239–246.

13. Lund JT, Ehman RL, Julsrud PR, Sinak LJ, Tajik AJ. Cardiac masses: assessment by MR imaging. *AJR Am J Roentgenol* 1989;152:469–473.

14. Gomes AS, Lois JF, Child JS, Brown K, Batra P. Cardiac tumors and thrombus: evaluation with MR imaging. *AJR Am J Roentgenol* 1987;149:895–899.

15. Utz JA, Herfkens RJ, Heinsimer JA, et al. Cine MR determination of left ventricular ejection fraction. *AJR Am J Roentgenol* 1987;148:839–843.

16. Utz JA, Herfkens RJ, Heinsimer JA, Simakawa A, Glover G, Pelc N. Valvular regurgitation: dynamic MR imaging. *Radiology* 1988;168:91–94.

17. Bisset GS 3rd. Magnetic resonance imaging of congenital heart disease in the pediatric patient. *Radiol Clin North Am* 1991;29:279–291.

18. Gomes AS, Lois JJF, George B, Alpan G, Williams RG. Congenital abnormalities of the aortic arch: MR imaging. *Radiology* 1987;165:691–695.

19. Amparo EG, Higgins CB, Hricak H, Sollito R. Aortic dissection: magnetic resonance imaging. *Radiology* 1985;155:399-406.

6

Abdomen

INTRODUCTION

A diagnostic scan of the abdomen generally consists of a T1-weighted coronal sequence and T1- and T2-weighted axial sequences. Occasionally, breath-held gradient-recalled echo (GRE) or spoiled GRE (SPGR) and images in the sagittal plane are useful. To achieve a quality scan, close attention should be paid to the imaging parameters. In most cases, the field of view should be adjusted to include just the abdominal contents, i.e., "trimming" off most of the subcutaneous fat on the patient's sides. This produces an optimal image that completely fills the space allotted on the film. Often, the tendency is to use a field of view that is too large, producing an image on the film that is conspicuously small. Magnifying the image to fill the space on the film tends to result in a blurry appearance.

Respiratory compensation is essential when performing standard spin–echo sequences. Because GRE and SPGR sequences are not compatible with respiratory compensation, these sequences should be performed during breath holding whenever possible. Fast spin–echo (FSE) imaging can be performed without breath holding by increasing the number of excitations to average the effect of motion. Unlike respiration, which is periodic, bowel peristalsis is random motion. Artifacts from random motion are not reduced by the use of respiratory compensation or breath holding. To reduce peristalsis and its resulting artifact, the patient should fast for 4 hours prior to the scan. Some body imagers also advocate the admin-

istration of glucagon, but this has not been proved to be routinely useful.

Because of the superior tissue differentiation provided by standard T1- and T2-weighted sequences, intravenous contrast administration (gadolinium) is often not needed. It is helpful in some circumstances, however. When used, the dosage is calculated by the patient's weight, as in neural imaging.

Similar to computed tomography (CT), a systematic search pattern should be developed when interpreting an abdominal MRI study. It is often useful to put the images from the T1-weighted and the most T2-weighted sequence (second echo) directly adjacent. Each organ should be examined for size, shape, homogeneity, and signal characteristics. One search pattern is to examine independently the entire liver, spleen, adrenal glands, kidneys, pancreas, retroperitoneum (including vessels and adenopathy), bowel, and mesentery, finishing with the bones and soft tissues. By following such a systematic search, the chances of missing a significant abnormality are reduced.

LIVER AND SPLEEN

The size criteria for a normal liver and spleen on MRI are identical to those of CT. One such criterion states that, if the liver spans less than 12 cm in the right midclavicular line, it is of normal size. A span of 15 cm or greater indicates hepatomegaly. A hepatic size between 12 and 15 cm is indeterminate. The assessment of splenic size is more subjective. When splenomegaly is present, the spleen often appears globular, may extend greater than 14 cm in the craniocaudal dimension, or may extend significantly greater than 50% of the abdominal size in the anteroposterior dimension. The hepatic size and contour can change with disease processes. Cirrhotic livers tend to have lobular instead of smooth margins and, often, have relative enlargement of the caudate and lateral segment of the left lobe.

Normally, the liver and spleen are slightly hyperintense to muscle on T1 weighting. The liver decreases and the spleen increases in signal intensity on T2-weighted sequences (Fig. 1). At 1.5 T, the normal T2 relaxation time (the reciprocal of T2, a quantitative means of evaluating relative T2-weighted signals) of the liver is approximately 45 to 55 msec. In hemolytic diseases, especially when a history of multiple

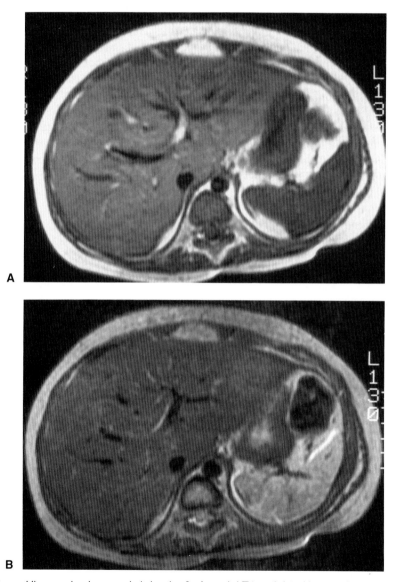

FIG. 1. Normal liver and spleen and cirrhosis. **A:** An axial T1-weighted image demonstrates the normal liver and spleen to be smooth in contour and slightly hyperintense to muscle. **B:** A T2-weighted image shows a loss of signal within the liver and an increased splenic signal.

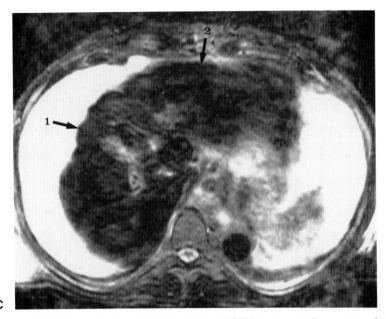

FIG. 1. *(continued)* **C:** Cirrhosis. An axial T2-weighted FSE fat-saturated sequence demonstrates a lobular hepatic contour (*1*) outlined by hyperintense ascites. Over all, the liver is shrunken in size, with the lateral segment of the left hepatic lobe being relatively enlarged (*2*).

blood transfusions is present, the liver, spleen, and bone marrow contain increased iron stores. The magnetic susceptibility of iron causes a decrease in the T2 relaxation time. In these cases, the liver, spleen, and bone marrow become visibly darker on T2-weighted sequences. The hemochromatosis associated with cirrhosis can result in an increase in hepatic iron stores, while sparing the spleen. A low-signal-intensity liver is seen in these cases, but unlike the iron overload of hemolytic anemias, the spleen often retains its normal high-intensity T2-weighted signal (Fig. 2). Some success has been reported in following hepatic iron stores using calculated T2 relaxation times rather than resorting to hepatic biopsy.

Fatty infiltration of the liver is associated with numerous processes, including alcoholism, obesity, diabetes, and hyperalimentation. It may be focal or involve the liver diffusely. Occasionally, it may simulate an infiltrating hepatic tumor but is usually much less conspicuous on T2-weighted images. Unlike a tumor, fatty infiltration does not alter the course or caliber of the hepatic vessels. The presence of fat can

be demonstrated by imaging the liver with a nonspin–echo technique, such as GRE. Two sequences are performed, each imaging the same region of the liver. The echo time is chosen appropriately, such that the fat and water are in phase for one sequence and out of phase for the other (see Chapter 1). When fatty infiltration is present, the involved portion of the liver will have a lower signal intensity in the out-of-phase compared with the in-phase sequence. Fat saturation sequences may also be helpful.

The segmental anatomy of the liver is defined by the venous anatomy. In general, the hepatic veins travel between lobes and segments, and the portal veins enter the segments centrally. The middle hepatic vein separates the right and left hepatic lobes, defining the interlobar fissure. The gallbladder also arises within the interlobar fissure. The right hepatic vein separates the right lobe into anterior and posterior segments; the left hepatic vein, traveling within the fissure for the ligamentum teres, separates the medial and lateral segments of the left lobe (Fig. 3). Using the venous anato-

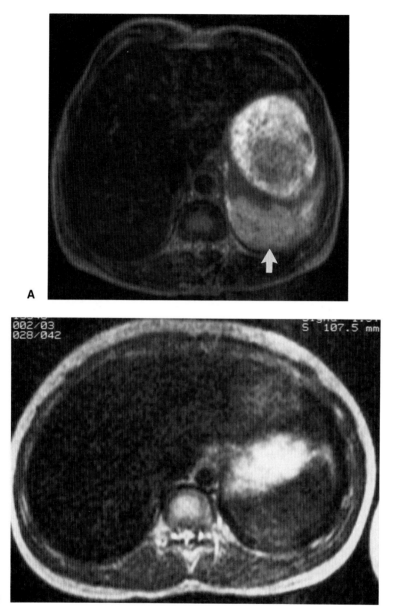

FIG. 2. Increased iron stores by axial T2-weighted images. **A:** Hemochromatosis. The liver is marked-ly hypointense, which is consistent with increased iron stores, but the spleen (*arrow*) is spared and retains its normal hyperintensity. **B:** Hemosiderosis. Both the liver and spleen are hypointense be-cause of increased iron stores in this 11-year-old patient with hemolytic anemia and a history of mul-tiple blood transfusions.

my to localize hepatic lesions is useful when surgical resection is contemplated.

The intrahepatic bile ducts travel with the portal venous branches and, when normal in caliber, are usually not seen. Dilated ducts pre-sent as linear structures that have a low signal intensity on T1-weighted and are bright on T2-weighted sequences (isointense with the gall-bladder).

An evaluation of space-occupying lesions is the most common indication for MRI of the liver. The sensitivity for their detection with

MRI (98%) slightly exceeds that of contrast-enhanced CT (93%). In addition, MRI provides an alternative to CT for establishing the diagnosis of a cavernous hemangioma. The ability to differentiate a hemangioma from a metastasis has important clinical implications because the latter situation often means a stage 4 malignancy whereas the former is a normal variant that occurs in up to 5% of the general population. The histological diagnosis of a hemangioma by needle biopsy can be difficult because the specimen often contains mostly blood, leaving some doubt as to whether the needle actually missed the cellular portion of a malignancy.

A cavernous hemangioma can be diagnosed with reasonable confidence by MRI if the lesion is homogeneous on both T1-weighted (dark) and T2-weighted (bright) images, round or oval in shape, sharply marginated, and has a T2 relaxation time greater than 88 msec. If the other conditions are met and the T2 relaxation time is less than 88 msec, the diagnosis becomes equivocal. Metastases, by contrast, tend be poorly marginated and may have a peripheral zone of increased or decreased intensity (halo sign). They are usually inhomogeneous centrally and less intense on T2-weighted sequences (T2 relaxation time less than 88 msec, often less than 60 msec, Fig. 4). The gallbladder can act as a gross internal control. Hemangiomas typically appear grossly isointense to bile; metastases typically appear hypointense on T2-weighted sequences.

Certain pitfalls in the diagnosis of hemangiomas should be considered. Multiple lesions are common with both metastases and hemangiomas, making multiplicity a poor discriminator. Giant hemangiomas (lesions greater than 4 cm) can also present a diagnostic problem because internal septations and heterogeneity are common. Simple hepatic cysts often fit the diagnostic criteria for hemangiomas on MRI. If this error is made, it is irrelevant to patient care because both lesions are generally benign, asymptomatic processes. Follow-up ultrasonography can reliably confirm a cyst. Cystic metastases or hepatic abscesses can have long T2 relaxation times but are usually associated with lesional heterogeneity.

The specificity for the diagnosis of a hemangioma is improved by a dynamic scan through the lesion during an intravenous bolus of gadolinium. Using a multiplanar SPGR or fast SPGR sequence gives a relatively T1-weighted image, and this can be rapidly performed and repeated in rapid sequence. The criteria for diagnosis of an hemangioma are the same as those for a single-station dynamic contrast-enhanced CT scan. The enhancement of the lesion begins in the arterial phase at the lesion's periphery, forming contrast puddles. As time progresses, lesions tend to fill in with contrast by central extension of the peripheral enhancement. There are disadvantages of this technique compared with an evaluation of a lesion by morphology and T2 relaxation time. The major disadvantages are the expense of gadolinium and occasional difficulty in evaluating multiple lesions during a single examination.

Focal nodular hyperplasia and hepatic adenomas are benign hepatic lesions. Because they may present with variable signal characteristics and heterogeneity, differentiation between the two lesions and from hepatocellular carcinoma may be difficult. The presence of a central scar is often seen in focal nodular hyperplasia, but it is not a particularly useful discriminator because it also may be present in adenomas and carcinomas (Fig. 5).

Hepatocellular carcinoma may present as a solitary mass, multiple masses, or diffuse hepatic infiltration. The lesions tend to be inhomogeneous. The signal characteristics tend to be variably decreased compared with normal liver on T1-weighted and increased on T2-weighted sequences (Fig. 6). In a cirrhotic liver, hepatocellular carcinoma can often be differentiated from a regenerating nodule by the former's increased signal on T2-weighted images. A regenerating nodule is often hypointense to normal liver. For a hyperintense lesion, a biopsy is needed to establish the diagnosis of hepatocellular carcinoma, but associated thrombosis of the portal or hepatic veins is highly suggestive.

The sensitivity of MRI for the detection of splenic lesions by standard sequences is limited. This is because the typical signal charac-

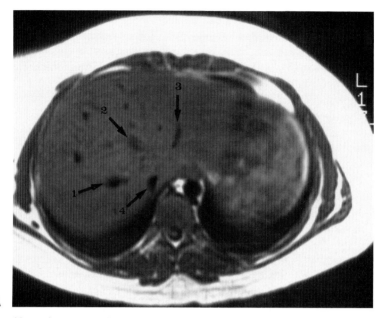

A

FIG. 3. Normal hepatic anatomy by axial T1-weighted images. **A:** Cephalad slice demonstrates the right (*1*), middle (*2*), and left (*3*) hepatic veins and the inferior vena cava (*4*).

teristics of many tumors are similar to the normal splenic signal (low-signal-intensity T1 and high-signal-intensity T2).

ADRENAL GLANDS

The normal adrenal glands generally are easily visualized on MRI and CT because of the presence of surrounding fat. Morphologically, they have a central body with two limbs forming an inverted V shape. On MRI, the adrenal glands are low to intermediate in signal on both T1- and T2-weighted images, being nearly isointense with muscle (Fig. 7). The sensitivity of MRI and CT are equivalent for the detection of adrenal masses; MRI has the advantage of multiplanar imaging (important in evaluating adjacent organ invasion) and the ability to differentiate some benign adenomas from malignant lesions by signal characteristics.

Biochemically active adrenal adenomas are uncommon, clinically symptomatic lesions. Their presence is actively sought by imaging studies, and when found, they are surgically removed. Biochemically inactive adrenal adenomas are found in 1% of the population. They

are clinically silent, often smaller than 3 cm in size, and are usually incidental findings on ultrasonography, CT, or MRI. Many of these incidental adenomas can be differentiated from adrenal carcinomas or metastases by signal characteristics, making a biopsy unnecessary. Adrenal adenomas typically have a calculated T2 relaxation time less than 60 msec; carcinomas and metastases have a relaxation time of greater than 60 msec (Fig. 8). Because bilateral adenomas are rare, bilateral adrenal masses strongly suggest metastatic disease.

Neuroblastoma is a childhood tumor that usually arises in an adrenal gland but may arise anywhere along the sympathetic chains (see Chapter 5, Fig. 5). It presents as a high-signal-intensity mass on T2-weighted sequences and metastasizes early (to the lymph nodes and bones). Calcifications occur 50% of the time. A GRE sequence can help in its detection ("blooming artifact"), but CT is more sensitive for the detection of calcification.

KIDNEYS

In general, CT is preferred over MRI for routine evaluation of the kidneys because of its

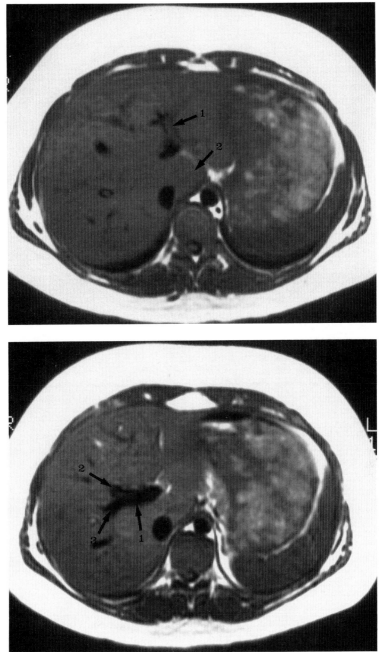

FIG. 3. *(continued)* **B:** Moving caudally, the left portal vein (*1*) and the caudate lobe of the liver (*2*) are seen. **C:** Progressing further in the caudal direction demonstrates the right portal vein (*1*) with its anterior (*2*) and posterior (*3*) segmental branches.

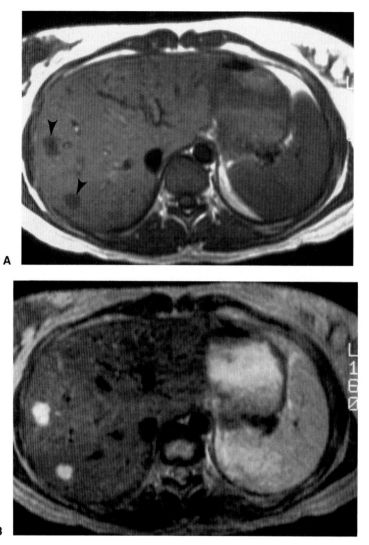

A

B

FIG. 4. Liver hemangiomas and metastases. **A:** Hemangioma. The axial T1-weighted image demonstrates two well-defined homogeneous space-occupying lesions (*arrows*) within the right hepatic lobe. **B:** T2-weighted image demonstrates the lesions to be sharply marginated and homogeneously hyperintense (the calculated T2 relaxation was 102 msec).

high sensitivity in detecting calcifications and perinephric disease. It is also less motion sensitive than is MRI. In patients who are allergic to iodinated contrast or in whom the CT findings are equivocal, MRI is an excellent adjunct in kidney evaluation. The multiplanar imaging capabilities of MRI can also be useful in determining the organ of origin for large masses projecting into the renal fossae.

Normal adult kidneys range from 9 to 14 cm in craniocaudal dimension. Corticomedullary differentiation is seen on T1-weighted images. The renal medullae is nearly isointense with muscle; the cortex is slightly hyperintense. On T2-weighted sequences, the renal cortex and medulla become isointense and high in signal intensity (bright, Fig. 9). Because these signal characteristics are similar to those of many renal cell carcinomas, detection of small lesions by standard spin–echo sequences can be difficult, especially when they are smaller than 3 cm. The use of gadolinium enhancement and

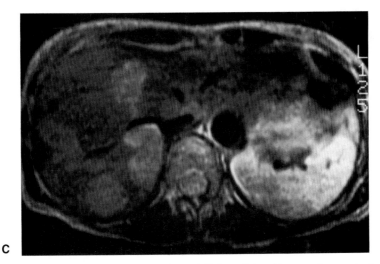

C

FIG. 4. *(continued)* **C:** Metastases (colon). An axial T2-weighted image demonstrates multiple hepatic masses, which are mildly hyperintense to liver (T2 relaxation times were 60 to 65 msec). The lesions are mostly homogeneous with well-defined margins, a somewhat unusual finding for metastases.

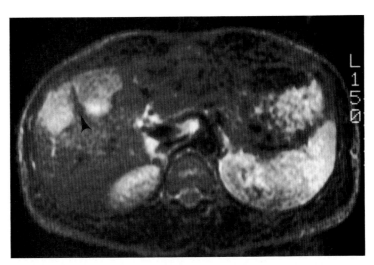

FIG. 5. Hepatic adenoma. The axial T2-weighted image demonstrates a moderately hyperintense hepatic lesion with some internal heterogeneity and a central scar (*arrow*). The presence of a scar suggests focal nodular hyperplasia, but the histological result was an hepatic adenoma.

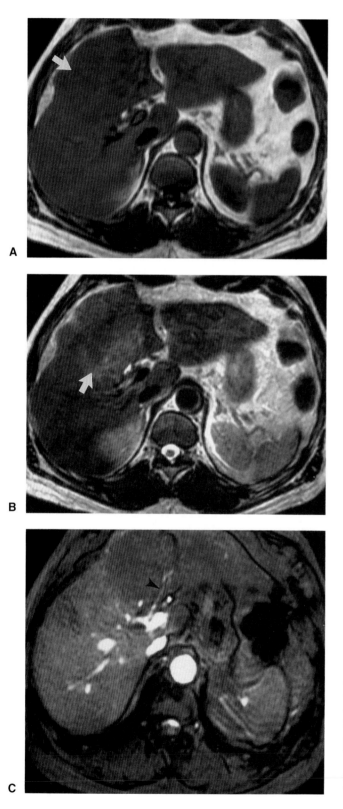

FIG. 6. Hepatocellular carcinoma. **A:** An axial T1-weighted image demonstrates the relative hypointensity of the left hepatic lobe compared with the right. The medial segment of the left lobe (*arrow*) also appears somewhat expanded, which suggests the presence of a mass. **B:** T2 weighting demonstrates an ill-defined, mildly hyperintense mass (*arrow*) in the medial segment of the left hepatic lobe. **C:** An axial GRE sequence demonstrates tumor encasement of the left portal vein (*arrow*) just distal to the porta hepatis. The portal venous branch extending into the lateral segment of the left lobe shows no high signal flow, which is consistent with thrombosis.

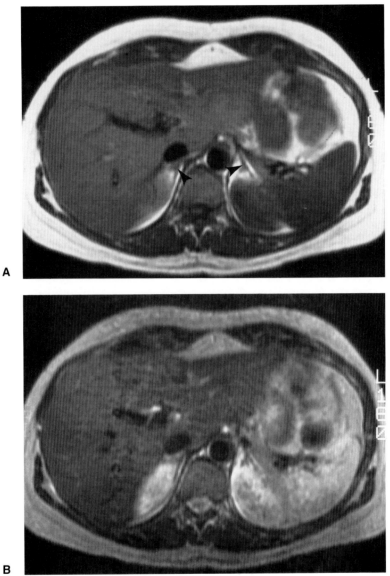

FIG. 7. Normal adrenal glands. **A:** An axial T1-weighted image shows a normal intermediate-intensity signal, with inverted V-shaped adrenal glands (*arrows*) surrounded by hyperintense fat. **B:** A T2-weighted image shows the adrenal glands remaining intermediate in regard to signal intensity.

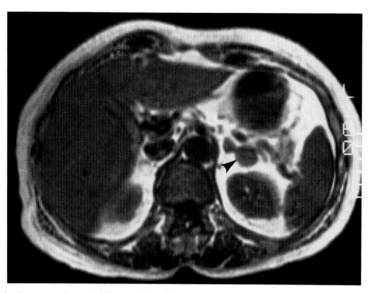

FIG. 8. Adrenal adenoma. An axial T1-weighted image reveals a rounded right adrenal mass (*arrow*). A T2-weighted sequence (not shown) demonstrated a T2 relaxation time of 52 msec, which is consistent with a benign adenoma.

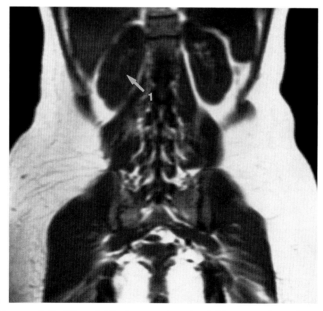

FIG. 9. Normal kidneys. **A,B:** T1-weighted coronal and axial images show the differentiation of the intermediate-signal medullary pyramids (*1*), from the renal cortex, which is slightly hyperintense. The normal pancreas is seen (*2*), following the course of the splenic vein (*3*).

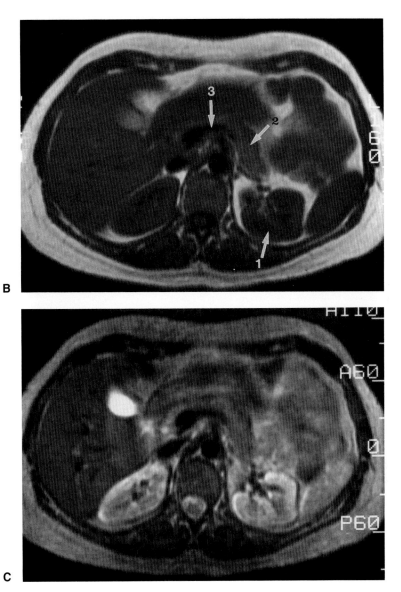

FIG. 9. *(continued)* **C:** An axial T2-weighted image demonstrates a relatively homogeneous renal hyperintensity. The pancreas remains intermediate in signal intensity.

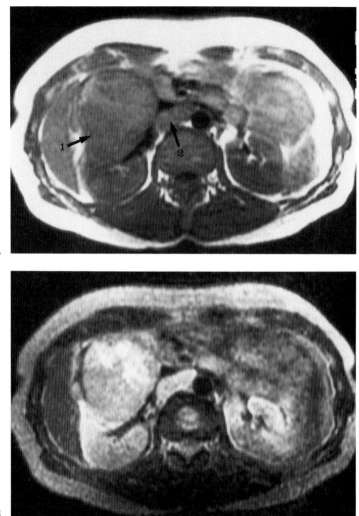

FIG. 10. Renal cell carcinoma. **A:** An axial T1-weighted image demonstrates a large renal mass (1), which is isointense to the normal renal parenchyma. Associated retrocaval adenopathy (2) is also present. **B:** A T2-weighted image demonstrates the hyperintensity of both the renal mass and the adenopathy. The mass remains isointense with the normal renal parenchyma.

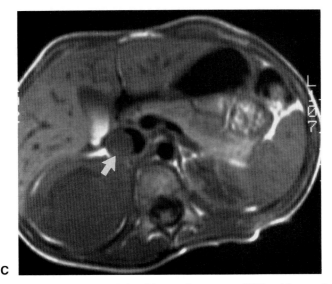

FIG. 10. *(continued)* **C:** An axial T1-weighted image in a case of Wilms' tumor demonstrates an example of vascular invasion. The tumor thrombus is present in the inferior vena cava (*arrow*).

fat saturation can improve the sensitivity for the detection of renal masses on T1-weighted (or SPGR) images. Gadolinium enhancement can also help to differentiate solid masses (enhancing) from renal cysts (nonenhancing) in equivocal cases.

In addition, MRI can stage renal cell carcinoma without the use of intravenous contrast material (Fig. 10). Vascular invasion presents as an intravascular mass on spin–echo images or as a signal void on GRE (flow-sensitive) sequences. Adjacent adenopathy is best seen on T1-weighted (low signal intensity) and T2-weighted (high signal intensity) spin–echo sequences. The presence of either vascular invasion or adenopathy indicates stage 3 disease. Invasion of adjacent organs (excluding the adrenal gland) or distant metastases indicates stage 4 disease.

An angiomyolipoma is a benign, solid, fat-containing, renal mass that can bleed and cause pain. Most commonly, they are seen in middle-aged women or in patients with tuberous sclerosis. The presence of fat within the mass is highly suggestive of an angiomyolipoma (Fig. 11), although a Wilms' tumor can also contain fatty elements. When hemorrhage is present, fat can be differentiated from blood products by the disappearance of the fat signal with a fat-saturated sequence.

PANCREAS

The pancreas follows the course of the splenic vein from the splenic hilum to the splenoportal confluence. It is typically intermediate in signal intensity on both T1- and T2-weighted sequences (Fig. 9B,C) Pancreatic carcinoma tends to be slightly hypointense on T1-weighted and often isointense with normal pancreas on T2-weighted sequences (not showing the marked increase in signal typically present with tumors elsewhere in the body). This makes small lesions difficult to detect. Furthermore, the contour of the pancreas may be obscured by motion from the overlying duodenum. Inflammatory pseudocysts can also be hidden by bowel undergoing peristalsis. Even though the use of gadolinium enhancement and fat-saturated breath-holding sequences improves a lesion's conspicuousness within the pancreas, MRI advantages over CT in pancreatic imaging may be limited to the lack of a need for iodinated contrast.

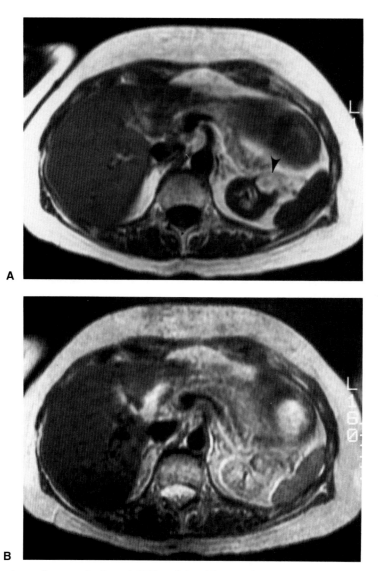

FIG. 11. Angiomyolipoma. **A:** An axial T1-weighted image demonstrates a right upper pole renal mass (*arrow*) that is isointense to the adjacent fat. **B:** The mass remains isointense to fat on T2 weighting.

ADENOPATHY

In general, adenopathy in the abdomen has similar signal characteristics to that of nodes elsewhere within the body. Typically, adenopathy is nearly isointense with muscle on T1-weighted and hyperintense on T2-weighted sequences (with a signal equal to or greater than that of fat). The nodes are considered abnormal by size criteria when they exceed 1 cm. It is not possible to predict the cause of adenopathy, whether it represents tumor or an inflammatory process, by the signal characteristics. Adenopathy can usually be differentiated from retroperitoneal fibrosis, which is typically low in signal intensity on both T1 and T2 weighting (Fig. 12).

ABDOMINAL AORTIC ANEURYSM

The normal abdominal aorta measures less than 3 cm in anteroposterior diameter, slowly

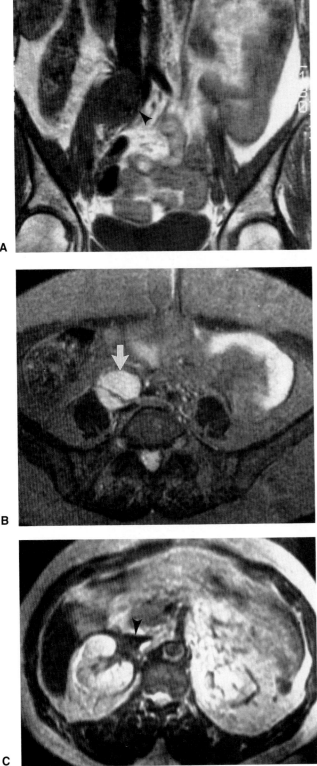

FIG. 12. Adenopathy and fibrosis. **A:** Adenopathy. A coronal T1-weighted image demonstrates a mass (*arrow*) that is isointense to muscle, adjacent to the right common iliac vessels. **B:** An axial T2-weighted image demonstrates hyperintensity (*arrow*), which is typical of adenopathy. **C:** Retroperitoneal fibrosis. An axial T2-weighted image demonstrates hypointense material (*arrow*) along the anteromedial aspect of the right kidney. The low intensity differentiates the fibrosis from adenopathy.

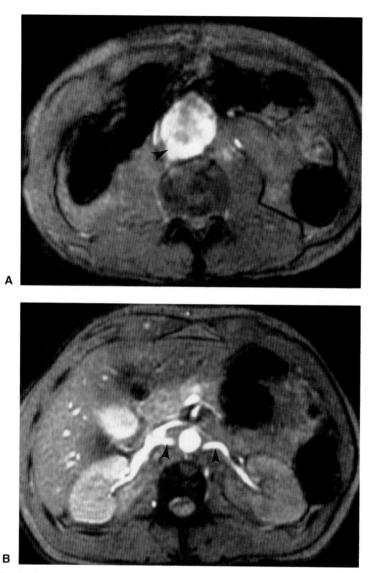

FIG. 13. Abdominal aortic aneurysms by axial GRE images. **A:** The bright signal indicates flowing blood within an abdominal aortic aneurism (*arrow*). **B:** Cephalad to the aneurysm, the aorta is normal in caliber. The renal arteries (*arrows*) are uninvolved.

decreasing in size to the bifurcation. Standard spin–echo sequences show fat abutting the aortic walls. Intraluminal flow void (low signal) is present on spin–echo sequences, although a high-signal-intensity central flow artifact may occur. The aorta is best evaluated by MRI in the axial plane.

An abdominal aortic aneurysm is present when the anteroposterior diameter of the aorta

exceeds 3 cm or whenever the diameter of the distal aorta exceeds the diameter of the aorta proximally. Surgical correction is often considered when an aneurysm exceeds 5 cm in the anteroposterior dimension. In their ability to measure aortic size accurately, MRI and CT are comparable. Without contrast, MRI can reliably demonstrate whether or not the aneurysm extends to the level of the renal arteries and to the aortic bifurcation (Fig. 13). This information is important to the vascular surgeon. The presence of mural thrombus can also be documented. T1- and T2-weighted spin–echo images are useful in detecting perianeurysmal blood products when leakage has occurred and in aging intraluminal thrombus.

BIBLIOGRAPHY

Books

1. Higgins CB, Hricack H, Helms CA. *Magnetic resonance imaging of the body.* 2nd ed. New York: Raven Press; 1992.

Journals

1. Kanzer GK, Weinreb JC. Magnetic resonance imaging of diseases of the liver and biliary system. *Radiol Clin North Am* 1991;24:1259–1284.
2. Mitchel DG. Focal manifestations of diffuse liver disease at MR imaging. *Radiology* 1992;185:1–11.
3. Gomori JM, Horev G, Tamary H, et al. Hepatic iron overload: quantitative MR imaging. *Radiology* 1991;179:367–369.
4. Thu HD, Mathieu D, Thu NT, Derhy S, Vasile N. Value of MR imaging in evaluating focal fatty infiltration of the liver: preliminary study. *Radiographics* 1991; 11:1003–1012.
5. Levenson H, Greensite F, Hoefs J, et al. Fatty infiltration of the liver: quantitation with phase-contrast MR imaging at 1.5T vs. biopsy. *AJR Am J Roentgenol* 1991;156:307–312.
6. Chezmer JL, Rumanick WM, Megibow AJ, Hulnick DH, Nelson RC, Bernardo ME. Liver and abdominal screening in patients with cancer: CT versus MRI imaging. *Radiology* 1988;168:43–47.
7. Lombardo DM, Baker ME, Spritzer CE, Blinder R, Meyers W, Herfkens RJ. Hepatic hemangiomas vs. metastases: MR differentiation at 1.5T. *AJR Am J Roentgenol* 1990;155:55–59.
8. Lee MJ, Saini S, Hamm B, Taupitz M, Hahn PF, Seneterre E, Ferucci JT. Focal nodular hyperplasia of the liver: MR findings in 35 proved cases. *AJR Am J Roentgenol* 1991;156:317–320.
9. Nokes SR, Baker ME, Spritzer CE, Meyers W, Herfkens RJ. Hepatic adenoma: MR appearance mimicking focal nodular hyperplasia. *J Comput Assist Tomogr* 1988;12:885–887.
10. Rummeny E, Weissleder R, Sironi S, et al. Central scars in primary liver tumors: MR features, specificity, and pathologic correlation. *Radiology* 1989;171:323–326.
11. Matsui O, Kayoda M, Kameyama T, et al. Adenomatous hyperplastic nodules in the cirrhotic liver: differentiation from hepatocellular carcinoma with MR imaging. *Radiology* 1989;173:123–126.
12. Hahn PF, Weissleder R, Stark DD, Saini S, Elizondo G, Ferucci JT. MR imaging of focal splenic tumors. *AJR Am J Roentgenol* 1988;150:823–827.
13. Baker ME, Blinder R, Spritzer C, Leight GS, Herfkens RJ, Dunnick NR. MR evaluation of adrenal masses at 1.5 T. *AJR Am J Roentgenol* 1989;153:307–312.
14. Kier R, McCarthy S. MR Characterization of adrenal masses: field strength and pulse sequence considerations. *Radiology* 1989;171:671–674.
15. Choyke PL, Pollack HM. The role of MRI in diseases of the kidney. *Radiol Clin North Am* 1988;26:617–631.
16. Hricak H, Thoeni RF, Carroll PR, Demas BE, Marotti M, Tanagho EA. Detection and staging of renal neoplasms: a reassessment of MRI imaging. *Radiology* 1988;166:643–649.
17. Semelka RC, Hrick H, Stevens SK, Finegold R, Tomei E, Carroll PR. Combined gadolinium-enhanced and fat-saturation MRI imaging of renal masses. *Radiology* 1991;178:803–809.
18. Steiner E, Stark DD, Hahn PF, et al. Imaging of pancreatic neoplasm: comparison of MR and CT. *AJR Am J Roentgenol* 1989;152:487–491.
19. Semelka RC, Kroeker MA, Shoenut JP, Kroeker R, Yaffe CS, Micflikier AB. Pancreatic disease: prospective comparison of CT, ERCP, and 1.5T MR imaging with dynamic gadolinium enhancement and fat suppression. *Radiology* 1991;1181:785–791.
20. Amis ES Jr. Retroperitoneal fibrosis. *AJR Am J Roentgenol* 1991;157:321–329.
21. Amparo EG, Hoddick WK, Hricak H, et al. Comparison of magnetic resonance imaging and ultrasonography in the evaluation of abdominal aortic aneurysm. *Radiology* 1985;154:451–456.

7

Pelvis

INTRODUCTION

The multiplanar capability and increased contrast resolution provided by T1- and T2-weighted sequencing make magnetic resonance imaging (MRI) preferred over computed tomography (CT) for the evaluation of many pelvic disorders. Because respiratory motion is minimal in the pelvis, high-quality images can be obtained without the use of respiratory compensation. The use of fast spin–echo (FSE) techniques produces superior image quality, saves time, and increases T2 weighting. The time saving is a key element because pelvic imaging often requires T2-weighted sequences in two planes (usually axial and sagittal). This is in addition to the standard coronal and axial T1-weighted sequences. The use of fat saturation is also compatible with FSE. Its use on T2-weighted images increases the sensitivity for the detection of tumor and inflammation (the high signal intensity from fluid is accentuated). To reduce the artifact from bowel peristalsis, the patient should fast at least 4 hours prior to the examination.

When evaluating MRI scans of the pelvis, it is useful to follow a search pattern to examine the patient systematically. This is facilitated by placing the T1- and T2-weighted axial images adjacent to one another so that morphology and signal characteristics can be evaluated simultaneously. One possible search pattern is as follows. Beginning at the aortic bifurcation, follow the common iliac vessels to their bifurcation; then, continue along the internal and external iliac vessels to the most inferior image. The

vessels should be evaluated for patency (intraluminal flow void). In addition, because lymph nodes tend to follow vascular chains, the presence of adenopathy is simultaneously sought. The obturator regions must also be examined (along the lateral pelvic walls at the level of the acetabuli) for lymph nodes. Starting at the anus and moving superiorly, the rectum, perirectal regions, and sigmoidal colon are then examined. If ascites is present, it is usually seen adjacent to the rectum because this is the most dependent portion of the peritoneal cavity in the supine position. The bladder's contour is then evaluated (coronal and sagittal images are helpful). The small bowel is examined, keeping in mind its margins are often obscured by motion artifact (peristalsis). The bones (marrow signal), musculature, and subcutaneous tissues are evaluated.

In a male patient, the prostate gland is then examined for size, zonal anatomy, and signal characteristics. Periprostatic tissues, including the seminal vesicles, are also evaluated. In the female patient, the uterus and cervix are screened for morphology and zonal anatomy. T2-weighted sagittal images are critical here. The ovaries should also be visualized and are best seen on axial images.

The sensitivity in detecting pelvic adenopathy by MRI is similar to that by CT. Lymph nodes in the pelvis are considered abnormal by size criteria when they exceed 1 cm in size. It is not possible to differentiate malignant from inflammatory adenopathy by signal characteristics. The appearance of adenopathy in the pelvis is similar to that of lymph nodes elsewhere in the body. Typically, the nodes are best seen on T1-weighted images as low-signal-intensity bodies surrounded by high-signal-intensity fat. On T2-weighted sequences, the lymph nodes generally become hyperintense to fat (Fig. 1). In difficult cases, gradient-recalled echo images with their inherent flow-related enhancement can differentiate vessels with slow flow from lymph nodes.

In general, MRI is preferred over CT for the evaluation of the pelvis for tumor recurrences involving the uterus, cervix, prostate gland, and perirectal region and during the postoperative and postradiation periods. Not only can a mass effect be detected, but the signal char-acteristics can help differentiate recurrent tumor (high T2-weighted signal) from posttreatment fibrosis (low T2-weighted signal, Fig. 2).

MALE PELVIS

The normal adult prostate gland weighs approximately 20 g. The prostate's size (in grams) can be estimated on MRI by multiplying length × width × height (each in centimeters) and dividing by 2. On T1-weighted images, the normal prostate appears homogeneous and intermediate in signal intensity (similar to muscle). On T2-weighted images, the zonal anatomy of the prostate gland becomes apparent.

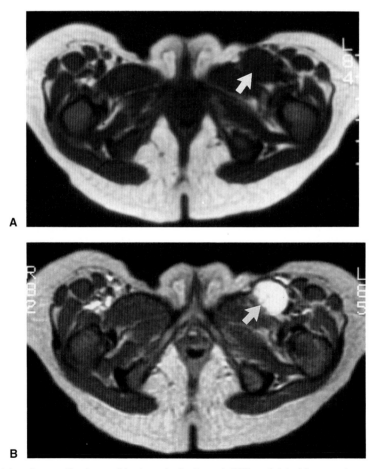

FIG. 1. Pelvic adenopathy (neuroblastoma). **A:** An axial T2-weighted image demonstrates a large left inguinal mass (*arrow*), which is isointense with muscle. **B:** An axial T2-weighted image shows typical hyperintensity of the enlarged lymph node.

The central and transitional zones are positioned anterior and centrally. They are low in signal intensity and are isointense to each other. The surrounding peripheral zone is high in signal intensity on T2-weighted images. It is bounded by the thin low-intensity fibrous capsule that surrounds the prostate gland (Fig. 3).

Benign prostatic hypertrophy (BPH) results from glandular proliferation in the transitional zone. As the gland enlarges, the volume of the transitional zone increases but maintains

its low signal on T2 weighting, although some heterogeneity with high-signal-intensity foci is common. The surrounding peripheral zone maintains its homogeneous hyperintensity but becomes a thin rim of tissue separating the enlarged transitional zone from the prostatic capsule (Fig. 4A).

Prostate cancer arises from the peripheral zone two-thirds of the time. The tumor tends to be lower in signal intensity on T2-weighted images than is the normal peripheral zone tis-

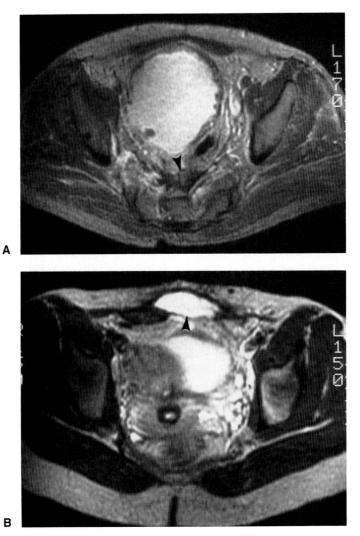

FIG. 2. Postoperative fibrosis *versus* recurrent tumor in axial T2-weighted images. **A:** Fibrosis. In a 61-year-old patient with colon cancer status postresection of a presacral mass, only low-signal-intensity fibrosis (*arrow*) is seen in the operative site. **B:** Recurrent tumor. The postoperative appearance of a hyperintense mass (*arrow*) in the anterior abdominal wall indicates recurrence of a desmoid tumor.

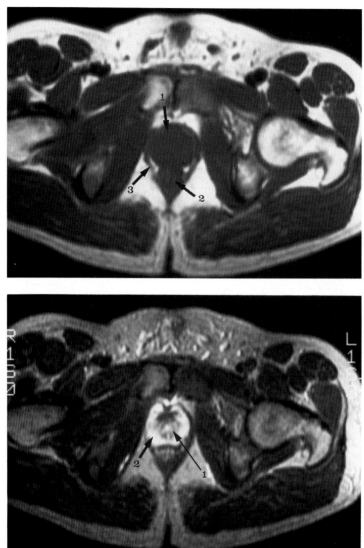

FIG. 3. Normal prostate gland. **A:** An axial T1-weighted image demonstrates a homogeneous prostate gland (*1*), which is isointense with muscle and bordered by hyperintense fat. The rectum (*2*) and levator ani muscles (*3*) are also seen. **B:** An axial T2-weighted image demonstrates normal prostate zonal anatomy. The central and transitional zones (*1*) are hypointense; the surrounding peripheral zone (*2*) is hyperintense.

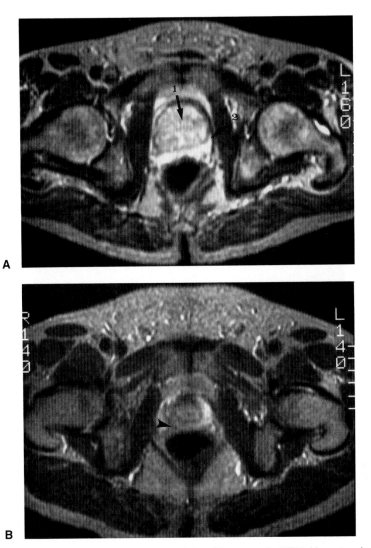

FIG. 4. BPH and prostate cancer in axial T2-weighted images. **A:** BPH. Hypertrophy of the hetero-geneously hypointense transitional zone (*1*) compresses the hyperintense peripheral zone (*2*) into a thin rim. **B:** Prostate cancer. The hypointense focus of tissue (*arrow*) within the normally hyperintense peripheral zone represents biopsy-proven cancer.

sue (Fig. 4B). This is somewhat unusual be-cause tumors elsewhere in the body are gen-erally hyperintense to their organ of origin on T2 weighting. Approximately one-third of prostate cancers arise within the transitional and central zones. Because of the normal tran-sitional zone heterogeneity in BPH, these tu-mors can go undetected by MRI until extension into the peripheral zone or out of the prostate gland occurs. Cancer often appears more ho-mogeneous than BPH, but on an individual basis, this is not a good discriminator.

Up to one-third of cancers within the prostate gland go undetected by MRI; therefore, the utility of MRI is not in diagnosing cancer but in staging the disease after the diagnosis has been made histologically. If the tumor is con-tained within the prostate capsule, Jewett stage A or B disease is present, and surgery becomes an option for cure. Whenever adjacent organ

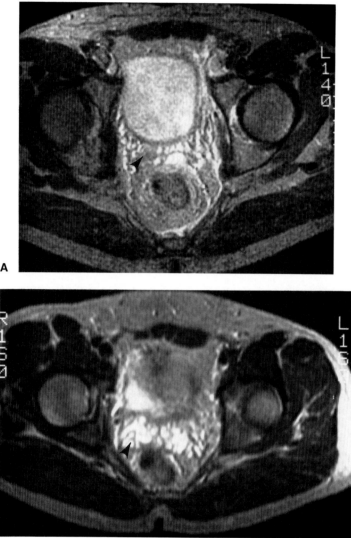

FIG. 5. Prostate cancer extending beyond the gland in axial T2-weighted images. **A:** The low intensity signal within the right seminal vesicle (*arrow*) indicates tumor involvement. **B:** Normal seminal vesicles are shown for comparison (*arrow*).

invasion (stage C), adenopathy, or distant metastases (stage D) are present (Fig. 5), treatment is restricted to radiation therapy.

Invasion of the seminal vesicles by prostate cancer constitutes stage C disease, and this can be accurately detected by MRI. The seminal vesicles are usually symmetric in size and located along the cephalad aspect of the prostate gland. They are normally multicystic in appearance and intrinsically high in signal intensity on T2-weighted images. When invasion by prostate cancer occurs, the normal high signal is lost, with the affected portions of the seminal vesicles becoming low in signal intensity (Fig. 5).

In addition, MRI can be useful in localizing undescended testicles. Localization for subsequent surgery is indicated because there is an increased risk of malignancy in cryptorchidism. Normal testicles are isointense to muscle on T1-weighted sequences and increase in signal on T2-weighted images. Axial scans through the lower pelvic cavity and inguinal canals should be performed when searching for an undescended testicle (Fig. 6).

FEMALE PELVIS

Uterus

In a nulliparous woman of menstrual age, the normal uterine size (including the cervix) is approximately 3 × 5 × 8 cm. Each dimen-

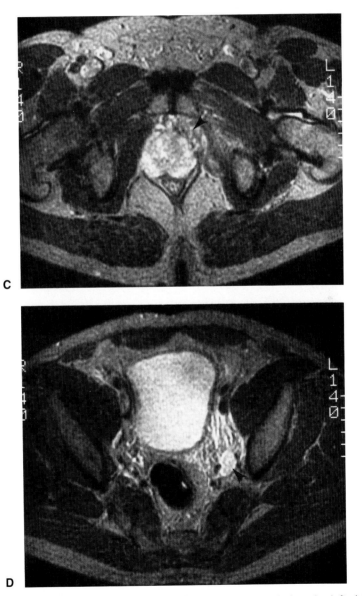

FIG. 5. *(continued)* **C:** Tumor extension beyond the prostate capsule into the left obturator internus muscle *(arrow)* is present. **D:** Adenopathy *(arrow)* in the left internal iliac chain indicates stage 4 disease.

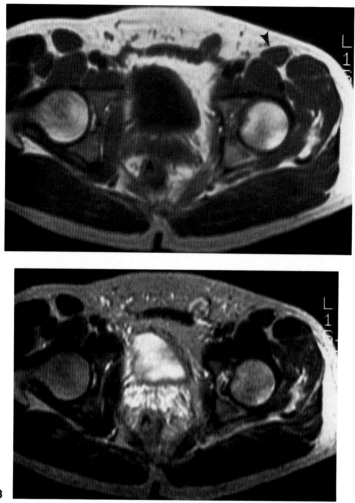

FIG. 6. Cryptorchidism. **A:** An axial T1-weighted image demonstrates a mass (*arrow*) that is isointense with muscle in the left inguinal canal. **B:** The mass (an undescended testicle) becomes hyperintense on T2 weighting.

sion may be 1.5 cm larger in a multiparous woman. The uterus can be subdivided into the corpus (body) and the cervix.

On T1-weighted sequences, the normal signal of the uterine corpus is homogeneously low to intermediate (isointense with muscle). Uterine zonal anatomy becomes apparent on T2-weighted sequences and, generally, is best evaluated on sagittal images. Three layers are identified: endometrial zone, junctional zone, and myometrium. Centrally lining the intrauterine cavity is the high-signal-intensity endometrium. Its short axis anteroposterior

thickness varies with the menstrual cycle but is usually less than 8 mm. Surrounding the endometrium and separating it from the intermediate-signal-intensity myometrium is the thin low-signal-intensity junctional zone (Fig. 7).

The uterine signal and endometrial thickness are dependent on the patient's hormonal status and age. With prolonged oral contraceptive use, the endometrium becomes thin and the junctional zone indistinct. A postmenopausal uterus also has a thin (narrow) endometrial zone and a decreased myometrial signal. If the patient

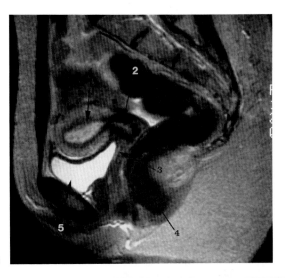

FIG. 7. Normal uterus and ovaries. **A:** A sagittal T2-weighted image demonstrates normal zonal anatomy of the uterine corpus and cervix. In the uterine corpus, the hypointense junctional zone (*1*) separates the central hyperintense endometrium from the peripheral intermediate-signal-intensity myometrium. The cervix has a thick hypointense stroma (*2*) around the high-signal-intensity mucosa. The vagina (*3*), rectum (*4*), and urine-filled bladder (*5*) are also seen. **B:** An axial T2-weighted image shows the uterus (*1*) and cyst-containing hyperintense right ovary (*2*). Free fluid (*3*) is also present in the cul-de-sac. **C:** An axial T1-weighted image demonstrates a homogeneous uterus and right ovary. Both are isointense with muscle.

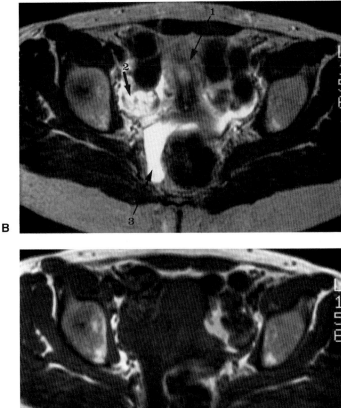

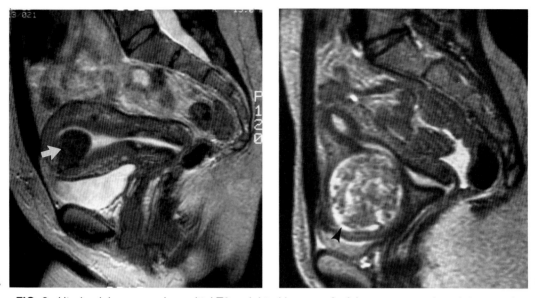

FIG. 8. Uterine leiomyomas in sagittal T2-weighted images. **A:** A homogeneous hypointense sub-mucosal fibroid (*arrow*) is seen projecting into the endometrial cavity. **B:** A heterogeneous degenerating intramural fibroid (*arrow*) causes mild distortion of the endometrial cavity without extension into the cavity itself. Despite the signal heterogeneity, the margins of the fibroid are well defined.

is receiving exogenous estrogen replacement, however, the uterine zonal anatomy appears identical to that of a menstruating woman. A premenarchal uterus is small in size and usually devoid of the high-signal-intensity endometrium.

Uterine leiomyomas (fibroids) are benign lesions that are commonly asymptomatic but may cause palpable uterine enlargement, dysfunctional bleeding, pain, infertility, and birth dystocia. Leiomyomas may be submucosal, intramural, or subserosal in location. Submucosal fibroids are the lesions most likely to be associated with bleeding and infertility. Myomas are isointense with normal myometrium on T1-weighted sequences and may be apparent only as a bulge in the uterine contour. On T2-weighted sequences, however, myomas are well-circumscribed masses, easily separable from any adjacent tissue. If no degeneration has occurred, myomas are homogeneously low intensity on T2 weighting (lower than myometrium). When degeneration has occurred, a heterogeneous increased signal is present within the myoma, but the margins remain well circumscribed (Fig. 8).

Adenomyosis is a condition in which endometrial tissue is contained within the my-

ometrium. The symptoms can be similar to those of uterine fibroids, including pain, bleeding, and uterine enlargement; MRI is a noninvasive means by which the differentiation of adenomyosis from leiomyomas can accurately be made. This is important because the treatments for the two disorders are different. Leiomyomas can be surgically removed with the preservation of the uterus (myomectomy), whereas treatment for adenomyosis requires a hysterectomy.

The myometrium may be involved diffusely with adenomyosis, causing widening of the uterine junctional zone, or it may present a focal mass. When focal, it typically is hypointense to normal myometrium on T2 weighting but may contain multiple punctate foci of high signal intensity. The margins of the lesion are indistinct with a wide zone of transition with adjacent myometrium. This is the primary characteristic that differentiates an adenomyoma from a leiomyoma (Fig. 9). Adenomyomas and leiomyomas may coexist within the same uterus.

Endometrial carcinoma for the most part is a disease of postmenopausal women. Clinically, it usually presents as painless vaginal bleeding. Because the signal characteristics are similar to those of the normal endometrium, the specificity for diagnosis by MRI is low. However, after the histologic diagnosis of endometrial carcinoma has been made (usually by dilatation and curettage), MRI is the imaging modality of choice for disease staging. One major advantage of MRI over CT is its ability to judge the depth of myometrial invasion. On T2-weighted images, when the tumor is confined to the endometrium, the endometrial layer may appear thickened, but the surrounding low intensity junctional zone will be intact. Interruption of the junctional zone by the high-signal-intensity tumor indicates myometrial invasion (Fig. 10). T1-weighted images with gadolinium enhancement may help in defining the depth of invasion.

The depth of myometrial invasion by endometrial carcinoma has prognostic implications. This is because, even though the tumor may appear confined to the uterus, (an Inter-national Federation of Gynecology and Obstetrics (FIGO) stage 1 lesion) increased depth of invasion is associated with an increased incidence of histological lymph node invasion. In FIGO stage 2 disease, there is cervical invasion; stage 3 disease is confined to the pelvis but has extrauterine extension. Stage 4 disease consists of rectal or bladder invasion or distant metastases.

Cervix

By contrast with the three anatomical zones seen within the uterine corpus on T2-weighted images, the normal uterine cervix has two. These consist of a central high-signal-intensity region (mucosa) surrounded by a low-signal-intensity stroma (Fig. 7A). Nabothian cysts are common benign processes consisting of dilated endocervical glands. They have a high signal intensity on T2 weighting (isointense

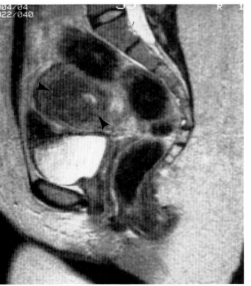

FIG. 9. Adenomyosis. A sagittal T2-weighted image demonstrates uterine enlargement. The hypointense junctional zone is widened. Unlike leiomyomas, low-signal-intensity adenomyosis (*arrow*) has poorly defined margins.

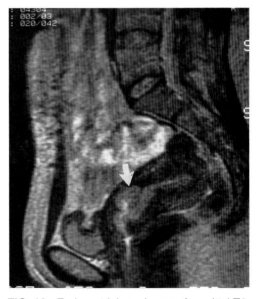

FIG. 10. Endometrial carcinoma. A sagittal T2-weighted image demonstrates a hyperintense mass (*arrow*) in the anterior uterine body. It crosses the junctional zone, invading deep into the myometrium.

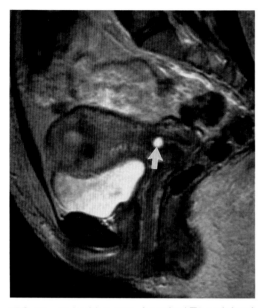

FIG. 11. Nabothian cyst. A sagittal T2-weighted image demonstrates a hyperintense, sharply marginated cyst (*arrow*) arising in the low-signal-intensity cervical stroma.

TABLE 1. *Differential diagnosis of an adnexal mass*

Physiologic cyst (follicular or corpus luteum)
Primary cystadenoma
Ovarian cancer
Metastases
Endometriosis
Dermoid
Pelvic inflammatory disease (tuboovarian abscess)
Ectopic pregnancy

with the endocervical canal), are sharply marginated, and extend into the low-signal-intensity stroma (Fig. 11).

Cervical cancer, like endometrial cancer, often presents clinically with vaginal bleeding. On MRI, it is high in signal intensity on T2-weighted sequences (isointense with the endocervical canal). Similar to endometrial cancer, the specificity for diagnosis of cervical cancer by MRI is low. After the histologic diagnosis is made, however, MRI is the method of choice in tumor staging. The major advantage of MRI is its ability to differentiate accurately FIGO stage 1 (tumor confined to the cervix and uterus) and stage 2A disease (extension to the upper one-third of the vagina) from more advanced disease. Stage 2A or less has the option of surgical treatment. Stage 2B (parametrial involvement), stage 3 (extension to pelvic walls or lower vagina), and stage 4 disease (bladder or rectal invasion or extension outside the pelvis) are treated by radiation therapy (Fig. 12).

For the evaluation of congenital uterine malformations, MRI is an effective method. The uterus is formed from the embryologic fusion of paired müllerian ducts. Abnormalities range from aplasia or hypoplasia to müllerian fusion anomalies, such as a bicornuate or didelphic uterus (Fig. 13). Associated unilateral renal abnormalities (usually aplasia) are common.

Adnexa

Ovarian size is best approximated as a volume (assuming a prolate elliptical shape) by the use of the formula: length × width × height (in centimeters) divided by 2. Ultrasound studies of normal ovarian size have suggested the following size criteria. Normal premenarchal ovaries average 3 cm³. The ovarian size increases through puberty. Young menstruating adults have normal ovaries averaging 10 cm³. Postmenopausal ovaries average 6 cm³. The ovaries are usually positioned laterally to the uterus, along the proximal external iliac vessels, but their location may vary. Normal ovaries have a low signal intensity (isointense with muscle) on T1 weighting and are hyperintense on T2. Because they may be isointense with the uterus and bowel on T1 and similar in intensity to fat and pelvic vasculature on T2, the ovaries may be difficult to identify unless ovarian cysts are present to help in their localization (Fig. 7). In menstruating women, the ovaries generally contain multiple physiological (follicular) cysts, each usually less than 2.5 cm in size, although an ovulatory cyst (corpus luteum) may be as large as 8 cm. Documenting the disappearance of large cysts after one to two menstrual cycles is useful in excluding malignancy.

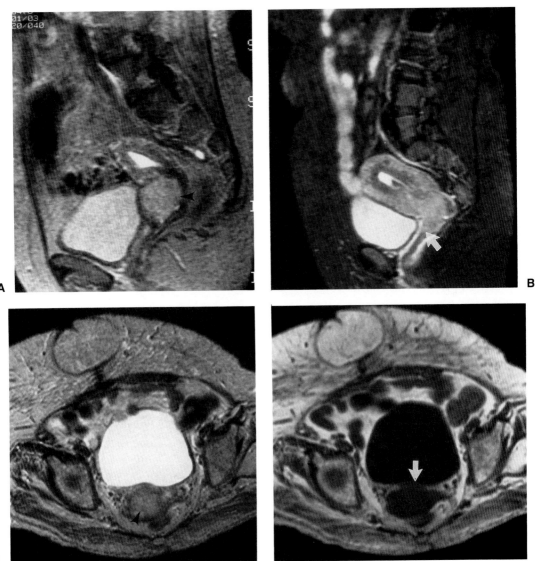

FIG. 12. Cervical cancer. **A:** FIGO stage 1 disease. A sagittal T2-weighted image demonstrates a relatively large, moderately hyperintense mass (*arrow*) confined to the cervix. **B:** Stage 2A disease. A sagittal T2-weighted image demonstrates a moderately hyperintense mass extending into the upper one-third of the vagina (*arrow*). **C:** Stage 4 disease. An axial T2-weighted image shows a moderately hyperintense cervical mass (*arrow*). **D:** The corresponding T1-weighted image shows extension of the low-signal-intensity tumor through the bright perivesicular fat to invade the bladder (*arrow*).

A useful differential diagnosis for adnexal masses is listed in Table 1. Some of the lesions listed can be adequately evaluated clinically and by ultrasound. MRI is useful in the diagnosis and preoperative staging of ovarian cancer. It is also helpful in diagnosing dermoid cysts and ovarian endometriosis.

Endometriosis results when foci of endometrial tissue are located outside the uterus. The most common sites of involvement are the adnexa and along the uterine ligaments, but endometriosis can be found elsewhere in the peritoneal cavity and within the retroperitoneum. The disease is often multifocal. On MRI, en-

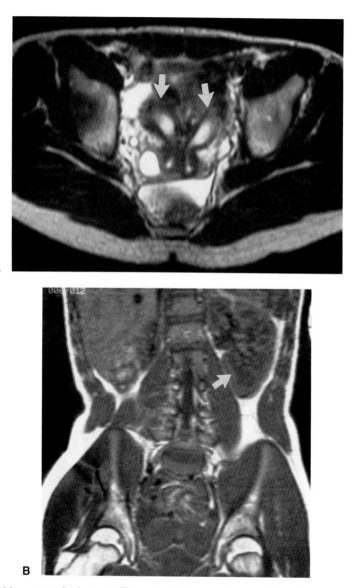

FIG. 13. Didelphic uterus. **A:** An axial T2-weighted image demonstrates two separate uteri (*arrow*) and cervices. **B:** A coronal T1-weighted image demonstrates a single kidney (*arrow*). Renal anomalies are often associated with congenital uterine abnormalities.

dometriomas may have signal characteristics identical to the uterine endometrial zone (dark on T1 and bright on T2). Contained blood products are common, resulting in high-signal-intensity components (methemoglobin) on T1 and, often, low-signal-intensity components on T2 (hemosiderin, Fig. 14). The presence of contained blood products and internal signal shading on T2 weighting helps in making the diagnosis of endometriosis. A surrounding low-signal-intensity fibrous capsule and adhesion to adjacent organs may also be present. Extraovarian disease is often underestimated by MRI because its presence is obscured by bowel peristalsis. As a result, laparoscopy remains the diagnostic procedure of choice.

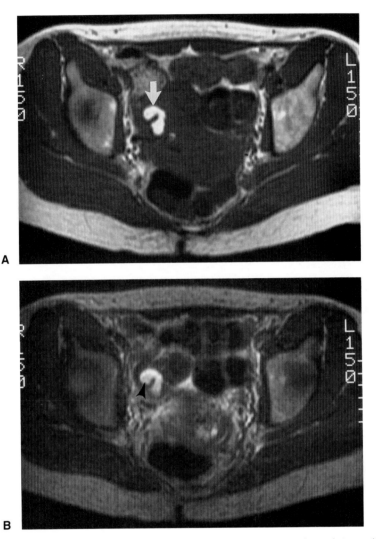

FIG. 14. Endometriosis. **A:** An axial T1-weighted image demonstrates hyperintense blood products (*arrow*) within a hypointense right adnexal mass. **B:** A T2-weighted image shows the signal intensity of the mass. The contained blood remains hyperintense but demonstrates some internal lower-signal-intensity shading (*arrow*).

The majority of ovarian teratomas are benign dermoid cysts. Characteristically, these lesions contain both a fatty component and a soft tissue mass (Rokitansky protuberance). Dermoids are bilateral in 15% of cases. The presence of fat within the mass, which is isointense to subcutaneous fat on T1- and T2-weighted images, is diagnostic (Fig. 15).

In addition, MRI is useful in evaluating ovarian tumors. Criteria have been developed to determine the likelihood of malignancy. These are based on five primary and four ancillary findings. The five primary criteria are size greater than 4 cm, large solid component, wall thickness of 3 mm, septa or nodularity greater than 3 mm thick, and necrosis. The four ancillary criteria are pelvic organ or sidewall involvement, peritoneal, mesenteric or omental disease, ascites, and adenopathy. When two

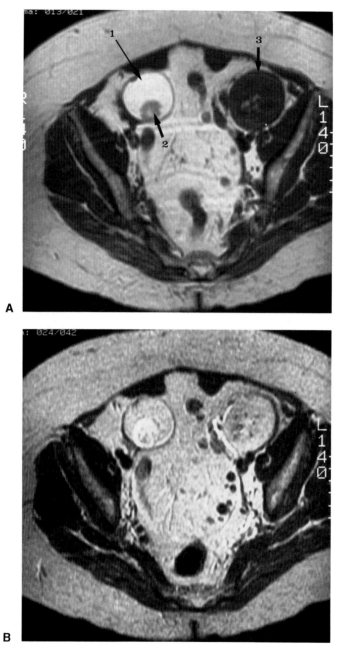

FIG. 15. Dermoid cyst. **A:** An axial T1-weighted image demonstrates a hyperintense mass (*1*), with a central hypointense component (Rokitansky protuberance, *2*), in the right pelvis. A low-signal-intensity transplanted kidney (*3*) is present in the left pelvis. **B:** A T2-weighted image shows the mass remaining isointense with fat. The Rokitansky protuberance becomes hyperintense.

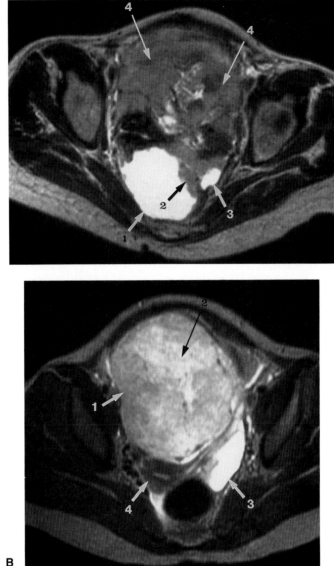

FIG. 16. Primary ovarian malignancy. **A:** Adenocarcinoma. An axial T2-weighted FSE image demonstrates a 5-cm cystic ovarian mass (*1*), with mural nodularity (*2*). Ascites is present (*3*), with diffuse studding and thickening of the mesentery (*4*). **B:** Malignant germ cell tumor. An axial T2-weighted image demonstrates a 10-cm mass (*1*), which arose from the left adnexa. It is primarily solid with a central cystic component or necrosis (*2*). Ascites is also present (*3*). The uterus is displaced posteriorly (*4*).

or more primary findings or one primary with one or more ancillary findings are present, malignancy is suggested (Fig. 16). If these criteria are not met, a benign process is suggested. The use of intravenous gadolinium enhancement improves the accuracy of diagnosis.

Most cases of ovarian cancer are already metastatic at the time of diagnosis; MRI can

be useful in staging the disease. The FIGO stage 1 disease is limited to the ovaries, stage 2 has pelvic extension, stages 3 has adenopathy or extrapelvic peritoneal implants, and stage 4 has distant metastases.

Metastases to the ovaries are usually from a gastrointestinal or breast primary. Ovarian involvement is typically bilateral. The lesions

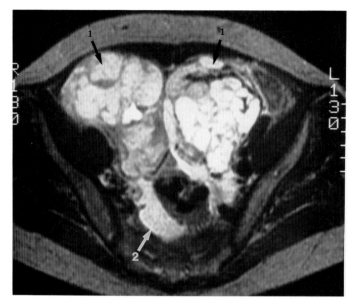

FIG. 17. Metastases to ovaries (colon). An axial T2-weighted image demonstrates large bilateral adnexal masses (*1*), which have cystic and solid components. Ascites (*2*) is also present.

may be solid or cystic. They generally have a low signal intensity on T1-weighted images and a high signal intensity on T2-weighted sequences (Fig. 17).

BIBLIOGRAPHY

Books

1. Higgins CB, Hricak H, Helms CA. *Magnetic imaging of the body.* 2nd ed. New York: Raven Press; 1992.

Journals

1. Nghlem HV, Herfkens RJ, Francis IR, et al. The pelvis: T_2 weighted fat spin-echo MR imaging. *Radiology* 1992;185:213–217.
2. Sugimura K, Carrington BM, Quivey JM, Hricak H. Postirradiation changes in the pelvis: assessment with MR imaging. *Radiology* 1990;175:805–813.
3. Hricak H, Dooms GC, McNeal JE, et al. MR imaging of the prostate gland: normal anatomy. *AJR Am J Roentgenol* 1987;148:51–58.
4. Allen KS, Kressel HY, Arger, PH, Pollack HM. Age related changes of the prostate: evaluation by MR imaging. *AJR Am J Roentgenol* 1989;152:77–81.
5. Carter HB, Brem RF, Tempany CM, Yang A, Epstein JI, Walsh PC, Zerhouni EA. Non palpable prostate cancer: detection with MR imaging. *Radiology* 1991;178:523–525.
6. Carrol CL, Sommer FG, McNeal JE, Stamey TA. The abnormal prostate: MR imaging at 1.5 T with histopathologic correlation. *Radiology* 1987;163:521–525.
7. Ling D, Lee JK, Heiken JP, Balfe DM, Glazer HS, McClennan BL. Prostate carcinoma and benign prostate hyperplasia: inability of MR to distinguish between the two diseases. *Radiology* 1986;158:103–107.
8. Biondetti PR, Lee JK, Ling D, Catalona WJ. Clinical stage B prostate carcinoma: staging with MR imaging. *Radiology* 1987;162:325–329.
9. Fritzsche PJ, Hricak H, Kogan BA, et al. Undescended testes: value of MR imaging. *Radiology* 1987;164:169–173.
10. Brown HK, Stoll BS, Nicosia SV, Fiorica JV, Hambley PS, Clark LP, Silbiger ML. Uterine junctional zone: correlation between histologic findings and MR imaging. *Radiology* 1991;179:409–413.
11. Haynor DR, Mack LA, Soules MR, Schuman WP, Montana MA, Moss AA. Changing appearance of the normal uterus during the menstrual cycle: MR studies. *Radiology* 1986;161:459–462.
12. McCarthy S, Tauber C, Gore J. Female pelvic anatomy: MR assessment of variations during the menstrual cycle and with use of oral contraceptives. *Radiology* 1986;160:119–123.
13. Demas BE, Hrick H, Jafee RB. Uterine MR imaging: effects of hormonal stimulation. *Radiology* 1986;159:123–126.
14. Togashi K, Ozasa H, Konishi I, et al. Enlarged uterus: differentiation between adenomyosis and leiomyoma with MR imaging. *Radiology* 1989;171:531–534.
15. Mark AS, Hricak H, Heinrichs LW, Hendrickson MR, Winkler ML, Bachia JA, Stickler JE. Adenomyosis and leiomyoma: differential diagnosis with MR imaging. *Radiology* 1987;163:527–529.

16. Hricak H, Stern JL, Fisher MR, Shapeero LG, Winkler ML, Lacey CG. Endometrial carcinoma staging by MR imaging. *Radiology* 1987;162:297–305.

17. Hricak H, Hamm B, Semelka RC, et al. Carcinoma of the uterus: use of gadopentetate dimeglumine in MR imaging. *Radiology* 1991;181:95–106.

18. Lien HH, Blomlie V, Trope C, Kaern J, Abeler VM. Cancer of the endometrium: value of MR imaging in determining depth of invasion into the myometrium. *AJR Am J Roentgenol* 1991;157:1221–1223.

19. Hricak H, Lacey CG, Sandles LG, Chang YC, Winkler ML, Stern JL. Invasive cervical carcinoma: comparison of MR imaging and surgical findings. *Radiology* 1988;166:623–631.

20. Kim SH, Choi BI, Lee HP, Kang SB, Choi YM, Han MC, Kim CW. Uterine cervical carcinoma: comparison of CT and MR findings. *Radiology* 1991;175:45–51.

21. Rubens D, Thornburg JR, Angel C, Stoler MH, Weiss SL, Lerner RM, Beecham J. Stage 1B cervical carcinoma: comparison of clinical, MR, and pathologic staging. *AJR Am J Roentgenol* 1988;150:135–138.

22. Carrington BM, Hricak H, Nurrudin RN, Secaf E, Laros RK Jr, Hill EC. M llerian duct anomalies: MR imaging evaluation. *Radiology* 1990;176:715–720.

23. Cohen HL, Tice HM, Mandel FS. Ovarian volumes measured by US: bigger than we think. *Radiology* 1990;177:189–192.

24. Olson MC, Posniak HV, Tempany CM, Dudiak CM. MR imaging of the female pelvic region. *Radiographics* 1992;12:445–465.

25. Arrive L, Hricak H, Martin MC. Pelvic endometriosis: MR imaging. *Radiology* 1989;171:687–692.

26. Ontwater E, Schiebler ML, Owen RS, Schnell MD. Characterization of hemorrhagic adnexal lesions with MR imaging: blinded reader study. *Radiology* 1993;186:489–494.

27. Togashi K, Nishimura K, Itoh K, et al. Ovarian cystic teratomas: MR imaging. *Radiology* 1987;162:669–673.

28. Kier R, Smith RC, McCarthy SM. Value of lipid-and-water-suppression MR images in distinguishing between blood and lipid within ovarian masses. *AJR Am J Roentgenol* 1992;158:321–325.

29. Stevens SK, Hricak H, Stern JL. Ovarian lesions: detection and characterization with gadolinium-enhanced MR imaging at 1.5 T. *Radiology* 1991;181:481–488.

8

Musculoskeletal System

INTRODUCTION

Magnetic resonance imaging (MRI) has virtually replaced arthrography for the evaluation of tendons, ligaments, and cartilaginous structures within and around most joints. Masses involving musculature or subcutaneous tissues also are often optimally imaged with MRI. Even subtle fractures are detected as a result of associated bone marrow edema. For the evaluation of cortical surfaces, complex fractures involving a joint, and some calcified lesions, computed tomography remains the imaging modality of choice.

Choosing the correct MRI sequence and imaging planes is important when designing a diagnostic study. The multiplanar capability of MRI is helpful in localizing and defining the extent of lesions. The bone marrow is evaluated on T1-weighted images and fat-saturated T2-weighted images. These optimize the contrast between the fatty marrow and fluid (edema or tumor) that may be present. The integrity of menisci of the knee is best evaluated with proton density images (long repetition time [TR] and short echo time [TE]), whereas ligaments or tendons may require more T2 weighting. Articular cartilage and joint fluid is generally well visualized on multiplanar gradient-recalled echo (MPGR) sequences. A gradient-recalled echo sequence best evaluates vascular patency. Masses require both T1- and T2-weighted sequences to define their extent and composition (e.g., fluid, hemorrhage, and fat). Fat-saturated T2-weighted fast spin–echo images may be particularly helpful.

KNEE

The knee is probably the joint most imaged by MRI. Because its anatomy is complex, it is important to develop a systematic search pattern for image evaluation. This ensures that each major structure has been examined. One such pattern is as follows. Beginning with a T1-weighted sequence (usually coronal), evaluate the bone marrow signal of the femur, tibia, fibula, and patella. A search along the joint's margins for osteophytes should also be performed. Articular cartilage is inspected on MPGR sequences (axial and radial sequences are suggested). The anterior (ACL) and posterior cruciate ligaments (PCL) and the quadriceps and patellar tendons are inspected on sagittal T2-weighted images. A joint effusion, which is a nonspecific finding of trauma or inflammation, is also best seen on this sequence. Medial and lateral collateral ligaments are then inspected on coronal images. Finally, the medial and lateral menisci are examined. This is best done on the proton density (first echo) of a T2-weighted sagittal sequence. A MPGR radial sequence, which views the menisci in an orientation similar to an arthrogram, may also be useful. Each meniscus is separately examined moving from the anterior horn to the posterior horn.

Occult fractures involving the distal femoral condyles or tibial plateaus can be seen on MRI. The apparent fracture line is the result of edema in the underlying bone marrow. Edema (water) has a low signal intensity on T1 (dark signal replacing the normally bright fatty marrow)

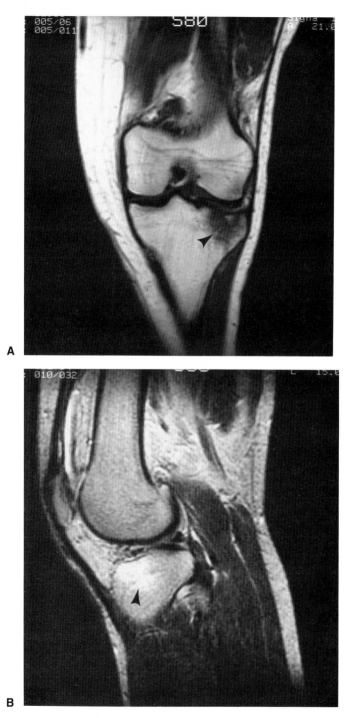

FIG. 1. Bone bruise. **A:** A coronal T1-weighted image demonstrates a region of low signal intensity involving the lateral tibial plateau (*arrow*). This represents marrow edema from a microtrabecular fracture. **B:** A sagittal T2-weighted image shows hyperintensity in the edematous region (*arrow*).

and is bright (slightly hyperintense to fat) on T2. It is best seen on fat-saturated T2-weighted sequences. When marrow edema is detected along an articular surface without a fracture being seen, a bone bruise (microtrabecular fracture) should be suspected (Fig. 1). Osteochondral disruption, such as osteochondritis desiccans, is also generally well seen (Fig. 2). This may result in a loose body within the joint (which may also be identified). Degenerative osteophytes often contain fatty marrow, which allows their visualization (Fig. 3).

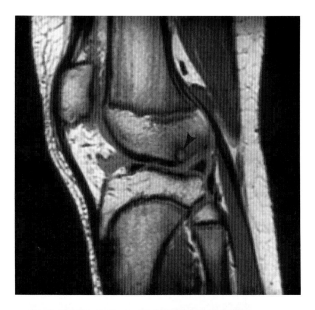

FIG. 2. Osteochondritis desiccans. A sagittal proton density image demonstrates a focal osteochondral defect (*arrow*) within the lateral femoral condyle.

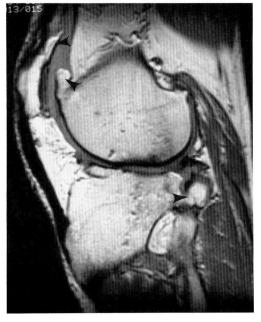

FIG. 3. Osteophytes. A sagittal proton density image demonstrates joint space narrowing and multiple osteophytes (*arrows*). The high signal intensity within the osteophytes represents fatty marrow.

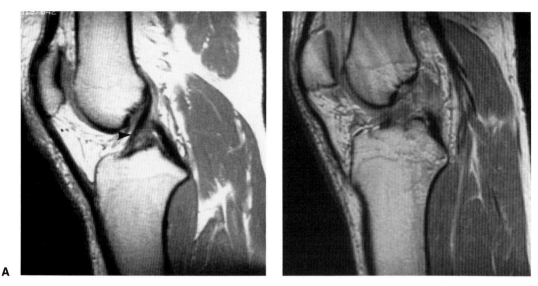

A

B

FIG. 4. ACL in sagittal proton density images. **A:** Normal ACL. Low-signal-intensity fibers (*arrow*) are seen in the intracondylar notch extending from the lateral femur to the medial tibial spine. **B:** ACL tear. No intact low-signal-intensity fibers are seen along the expected course of the ACL.

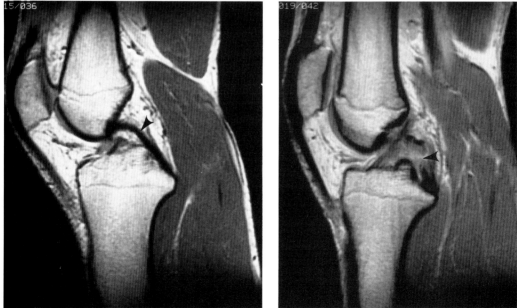

A

B

FIG. 5. PCL in sagittal proton density images. **A:** Normal PCL. Low-signal-intensity fibers (*arrow*) are seen in the intracondylar notch extending from the medial femur to the lateral tibial spine. **B:** PCL tear. High-signal-intensity disruption of the low-signal-intensity PCL is present (*arrow*).

The cruciate ligaments are optimally imaged on a T2-weighted sagittal sequence with the knee externally rotated 15°. Like other ligaments, they should be low in signal intensity on all imaging sequences. When a tear is present, an increased signal is seen along the normal ligamentous course. When the tear is complete, no intact low-signal-intensity fibers are seen in the region of the tear. Tears of the ACL are common (Fig. 4). A tear of the PCL is rare (Fig. 5).

A coronal view best demonstrates the collateral ligaments. The normal medial collateral ligament is composed of a band of

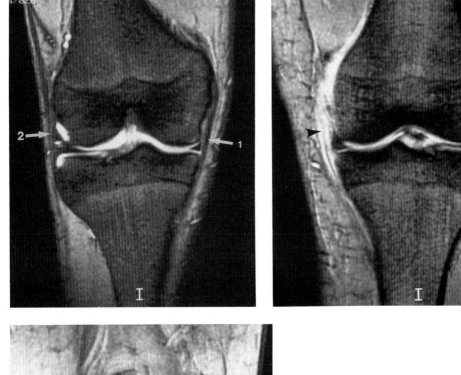

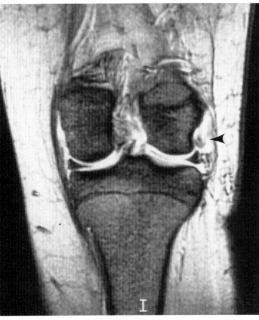

FIG. 6. Collateral ligaments in coronal MPGR images. **A:** Normal medial (*MCL*) and lateral (*LCL*) collateral ligaments. Intact low-signal-intensity fibers of the MCL (*1*) and LCL (*2*) are seen. **B:** MCL tear. No intact low-signal-intensity fibers are seen along the expected course of the MCL, instead a high-intensity signal (*arrow*) is present. **C:** LCL tear. Disruption of the LCL with a high-intensity signal (*arrow*) is apparent.

low-signal-intensity fibers that originate along the distal femur and attach along the proximal tibia. It also attaches to the medial joint capsule (which is attached to the medial meniscus). The normal lateral collateral ligament is more cord-like in configuration and attaches to the fibular head. No capsular attachment is present. When a tear of the medial collateral ligament is present, an increased signal intensity can be seen along the expected tendinous course (Fig. 6). Tears are best seen on T2-weighted sequences. A complete tear may be associated with medial meniscal and ACL tears. Tears of the lateral collateral ligament are uncommon.

Both the medial and lateral menisci are C shaped in the axial plane. They function to stabilize the articulation of the femur and tibia throughout complex knee motion. Because the menisci are fibrocartilage, they are low in signal intensity on all standard sequences. Menisci are optimally evaluated on proton density images (long TR and short TE) and MPGR sequences. Sagittal and radial images slice the menisci perpendicular to the long axis, resulting in a triangular appearance (similar to the arthrographic appearance). This plane is ideal for the detection of meniscal degeneration and tears.

The severity of meniscal degeneration can be graded by its MRI appearance. Except for differences in position, the findings of degeneration (and tears) are identical in both the medial and lateral menisci. Grade 1 degeneration demonstrates increased punctate or globular intrasubstance signal. Grade 2 has increased linear intrasubstance signal. The intrasubstance signal does not extend to an articular surface (edge the meniscus) in either grade 1 or 2 degeneration. Signal extension to the meniscal surface (superior, inferior, or meniscal apex) is the criterion for the diagnosis of a meniscal tear (also classified as grade 3 degeneration, Fig. 7). These tears are generally linear in configuration, but they may have a branching pattern of signal (complex tear). Meniscal maceration shows a diffuse increased signal intensity extending to both the superior and inferior articular surfaces (Fig. 8).

A horizontal tear along the long axis of the meniscus can result in a separation of the meniscus into two C-shaped fragments. One fragment can become displaced medially. This is called a "bucket-handle" tear. On MRI, the meniscal fragment in the normal anatomical position appears diminished in height. The displaced fragment can often be seen medially, within the intercondylar notch (Fig. 9). Two common pitfalls that can result in a false-positive diagnosis for a meniscal tear occur at the insertion of the anterior transverse ligament and at the insertion of the popliteal tendon. The transverse ligament traverses the anterior knee, attaching the frontal horns of the medial and lateral menisci. At its meniscal insertions, an obliquely oriented linear region of signal is sometimes seen. The insertion of the popliteal tendon (and sheath) into the posterior horn of the lateral meniscus has a similar linear region of signal (Fig. 10). Although both cases may mimic a meniscal tear, the linear signal is actually extrameniscal, separating the normal low-signal-intensity meniscus from the normal low-signal-intensity ligament or tendon.

SHOULDER

A routine shoulder MRI should include a T1-weighted sequence (to examine the bone marrow), a T2-weighted coronal oblique sequence (preferably with fat saturation to examine the rotator cuff), and an MPGR sequence (usually axial to examine the glenoid labrum). Four tendons surround the humeral head, inserting on the joint capsule to make up the rotator cuff. These are the supraspinatus, infraspinatus, teres minor, and subscapularis tendons (Fig. 11). Most injuries to the rotator cuff involve the distal supraspinous tendon in the "critical zone" (a relatively avascular zone approximately 1 cm from the humeral insertion site). These injuries may be associated with impingement on the subacromial space by hypertrophy of the acromion or acromioclavicular joint. Tendon injury from impingement (impingement syndrome) runs the spectrum from tendonitis and partial tear to complete tear of the rotator cuff.

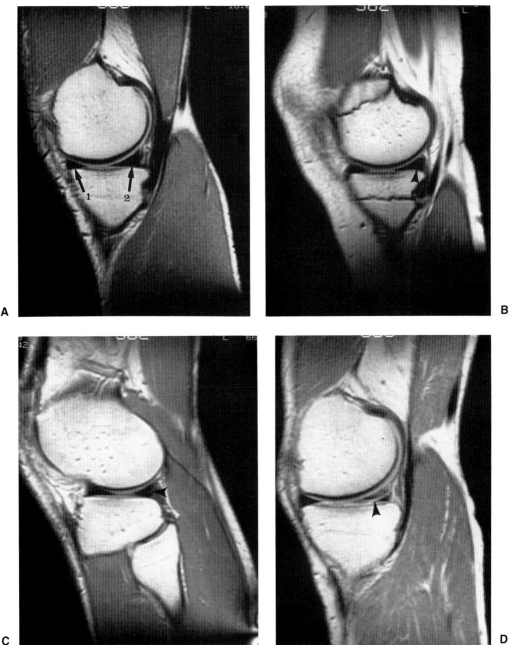

FIG. 7. Normal meniscus and meniscal degeneration in sagittal proton density images. **A:** Normal meniscus. The triangular anterior horn (*1*) and posterior horn (*2*) of the medial meniscus are homogeneously hypointense. **B:** A globular signal (*arrow*) within the posterior horn of the medial meniscus without extension to an articular surface indicates grade 1 degeneration. **C:** A linear signal (*arrow*) within the posterior horn of the lateral meniscus without extension to the meniscal surface represents grade 2 degeneration. **D:** A linear signal within the posterior horn of the medial meniscus extending to the inferior articular surface is diagnostic for a meniscal tear (grade 3 degeneration).

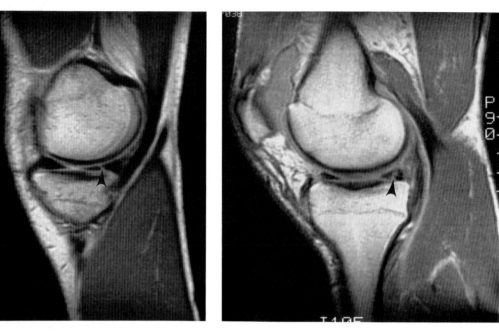

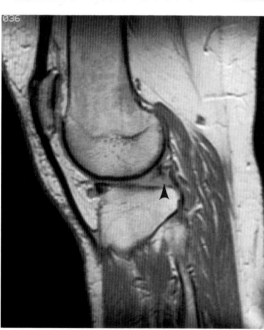

FIG. 8. Meniscal tears in sagittal proton density images. **A:** Linear (vertical) meniscal tear (*arrow*). **B:** Complex (branching) tear (*arrow*). **C:** Meniscal maceration (*arrow*). The posterior horn of the lateral meniscus shows a diffuse increased signal intensity that extends to both articular surfaces.

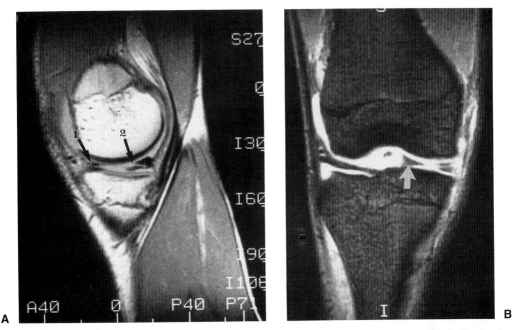

FIG. 9. Bucket-handle meniscal tear. **A:** A sagittal proton density image demonstrates diminution in the size of the anterior horn (*1*) and a horizontal tear (*2*) in the posterior horn of the medial meniscus. **B:** A coronal MPGR image shows meniscal material within the medial intracondylar notch (*arrow*), which is diagnostic for a bucket-handle tear.

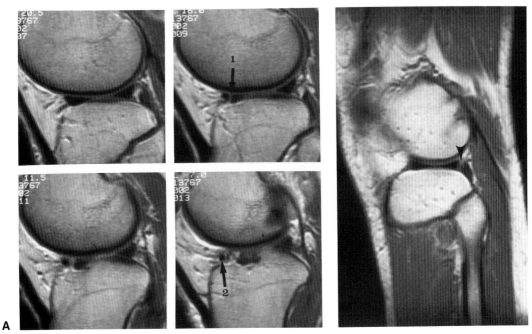

FIG. 10. Normal anatomy mimicking meniscal tears. **A:** Transverse ligament. A sagittal proton density four-on-one image demonstrates the appearance of a tear within the anterior horn (*1*). A section nearer the intracondylar notch demonstrates the suspected anterior meniscal fragment is in continuity with and actually represents the transverse ligament (*2*). **B:** A linear hyperintense signal (*arrow*) at the popliteal tendon insertion point into the posterior horn of the lateral meniscus can mimic a meniscal tear.

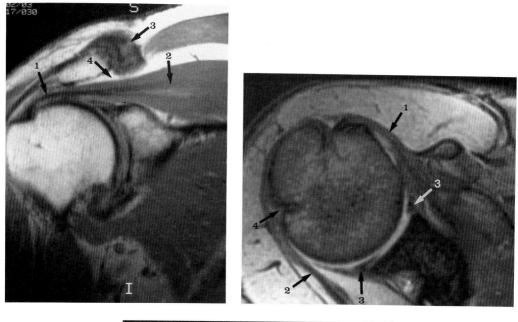

A

B

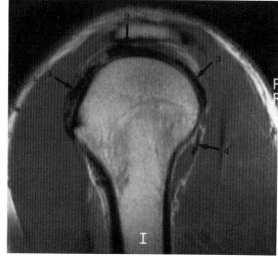

C

FIG. 11. Normal rotator cuff tendons. **A:** An oblique coronal proton density image demonstrates the entire course of the low-signal-intensity supraspinatus tendon (*1*), from its origin within the supraspinatus muscle (*2*), to its insertion near the greater tuberosity of the humerus. Low-signal-intensity hypertrophy of the acromioclavicular joint (*3*) is present, but the fat within the subacromial space (*4*) is preserved. **B:** An axial MPGR image demonstrates the normal low-signal-intensity subscapularis tendon (*1*) anteriorly and the infraspinatus tendon (*2*) posteriorly. The normal glenoid labrum (*3*) is also seen. A Hill-Sachs fracture deformity (*4*) of the humeral head is shown. This patient had a history of anterior shoulder dislocation. **C:** An oblique sagittal proton density image demonstrates the subscapularis (*1*), supraspinatus (*2*), infraspinatus (*3*), and teres minor (*4*) tendons encircling the humeral head to form the rotator cuff.

The criteria for a complete rotator cuff tear is met when an increased signal on T1-weighted (or proton density) images is seen to involve the entire thickness of the normally low-signal-intensity tendon. In addition, the high signal intensity within the tendon must persist on the T2-weighted sequence, being hyperintense to adjacent muscle (Fig. 12). These findings are usually best seen in the coronal oblique pro-jection. Sometimes, the supraspinatus tendon may appear completely disrupted with retraction and atrophy of the supraspinatus muscle. Adjunctive findings of a complete rotator cuff tear include fluid in the subdeltoid or subacromial bursa and diminished subacromial fat. Tendonitis and partial rotator cuff tears cannot be reliably differentiated from each other by MRI. They appear similar to a complete tear,

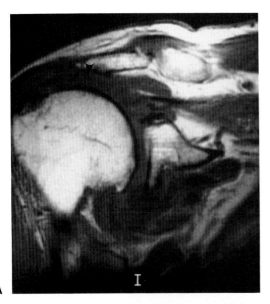

A

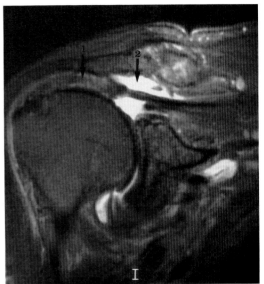

B

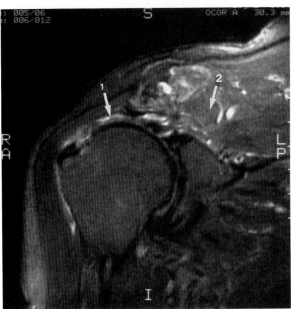

C

FIG. 12. Complete rotator cuff tear. **A:** An oblique coronal T1-weighted image demonstrates an intermediate signal intensity (*arrow*) involving the entire thickness of the normally low-signal-intensity supraspinatus tendon. **B:** A T2-weighted fat-saturated image shows a persistent signal increase within the supraspinatus tendon (*1*). Notice the absence of subacromial fat and the presence of fluid (*2*) within the subacromial bursa. **C:** An oblique coronal T2-weighted image in another patient demonstrates a high riding shoulder with complete disruption of the supraspinatus tendon (*1*). The supraspinatus muscle is retracted (*2*).

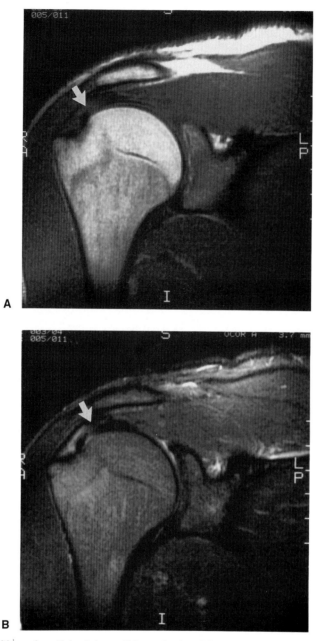

FIG. 13. Tendonitis and partial rotator cuff tear. **A:** An oblique coronal T1-weighted image demonstrates an intermediate signal intensity along the distal supraspinatus tendon (*arrow*). **B:** A T2-weighted fat-saturated image shows a persistent high signal intensity (*arrow*), but the entire tendon thickness is not involved (some low-signal-intensity fibers persist). This is consistent with a partial tear or tendonitis.

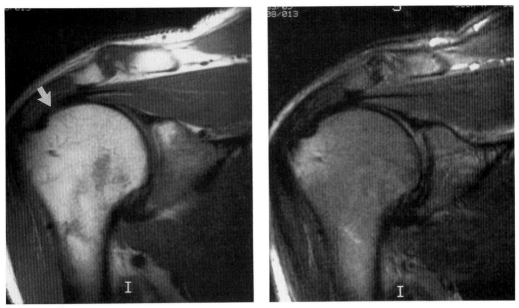

FIG. 14. Magic angle phenomenon, which mimics a rotator cuff tear. **A:** An oblique coronal T1-weighted image demonstrates an intermediate signal intensity within the distal supraspinatus tendon (*arrow*), suggesting a tear. **B:** A T2-weighted fat-saturated image shows the disappearance of the high signal focus. This indicates that the signal increase on the short TE (T1) image was artifactual. No tear is present.

except that the region of increased signal does not extend through the entire thickness of the low-signal-intensity tendon (Fig. 13).

Artifacts can mimic the findings of rotator cuff abnormalities on the T1-weighted and proton density images. The presence of a focally increased signal intensity within the supraspinatus tendon is seen on these sequences in some normal subjects. This artifactual signal may be caused by imaging that is done out of the plane of the supraspinatus tendon, allowing a partial volume of fat between the distal supraspinatus and infraspinatus tendons. Alternatively, the increased signal may be a result of a "magic angle" phenomenon. This is seen on short TE images when the tendon is aligned at a 45° to 60° angle in relation to the scanner's static magnetic field. True rotator cuff tears are differentiated from artificial signals in the supraspinatus tendon by use of a long TE (T2-weighted sequence). If the focus of signal increase persists on this sequence, a true cuff injury is present. An artificial signal resulting from the magic

angle phenomenon will disappear when using a long TE (Fig. 14).

The cartilaginous glenoid labrum is generally well seen on MPGR sequences. Labral tears usually occur anteriorly and are best seen in the axial plane. They appear as a high-signal-intensity defect in the normally low-signal-intensity triangular-shaped cartilage. A tear of the labrum may be difficult to diagnose, however, because of wide variation in the normal labral appearance. This limitation can be overcome by performing an MR arthrogram. Under fluoroscopic guidance, 10 ml of dilute gadolinium (0.4 ml or 0.2 mmol of gadolinium diluted in 100 ml of normal saline) is injected with 0.3 ml of epinephrine (1:1000) into the shoulder joint. Immediately following the injection, MRI is performed. The sequences should include T1-weighted images in the axial and oblique coronal projections. If a glenoid labral tear is present, the high-signal-intensity gadolinium will outline the defect within the low-signal-intensity cartilage (Fig. 15).

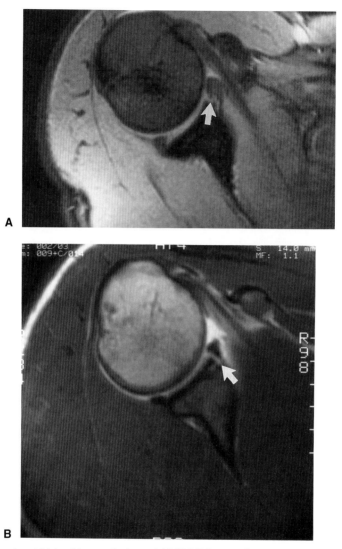

FIG. 15. Anterior glenoid labral tears. **A:** An axial MPGR image demonstrates avulsion of the labral cartilage from the glenoid (*arrow*). **B:** An axial T1-weighted image with intraarticular gadolinium demonstrates the high-signal-intensity gadolinium within a labral tear (*arrow*).

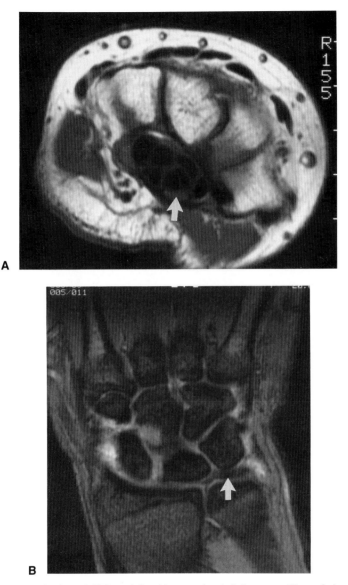

FIG. 16. Normal wrist. **A:** An axial T1-weighted image through the carpal tunnel shows the finger flexor tendons and the median nerve (*arrow*). **B:** A coronal MPGR image demonstrates the normal hypointense triangular fibrocartilage (*arrow*).

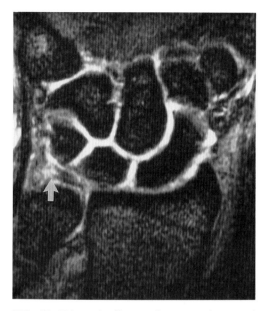

FIG. 17. Triangular fibrocartilage tear. A coronal MPGR image shows a high-signal-intensity disruption of the triangular fibrocartilage (*arrow*).

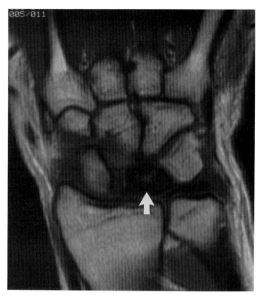

FIG. 18. AVN. A coronal T1-weighted image demonstrates a low-signal-intensity replacement of the normally hyperintense lunate marrow (*arrow*). This represents Kienböck's disease.

WRIST

With the use of a dedicated wrist coil, the integrity of the bony and ligamentous structures of the wrist can be evaluated. The carpal tunnel is best imaged axially; the triangular fibrocartilage and carpal ligaments are best imaged coronally (Fig. 16). An increased signal intensity within the normally low-signal-intensity triangular fibrocartilage indicates a tear (Fig. 17). Early avascular necrosis (AVN) following a carpal fracture can also be detected by the ensuing low-intensity marrow signal (Fig. 18). Fat-saturated T2-weighted images may show marrow edema best.

TEMPOROMANDIBULAR JOINT (TMJ)

Obliquely oriented sagittal T1-weighted images best demonstrate the relationship of the meniscus (disc) with the mandibular condyle. The meniscus is made of fibrocartilage and is normally low in signal intensity. It has a "bowtie" shape with triangular anterior and poste-

rior bands connected by a thin intermediate zone (Fig. 19A). The intermediate zone is normally positioned along the condyle at the point of closest approximation with the temporal bone articulation. When the mouth opens, the meniscus translocates anteriorly with the condyle to maintain this relationship.

Almost all meniscal dislocations are anteromedial. The diagnosis is made when the thin intermediate zone no longer maintains its normal relationship with the condylar articulation (Fig. 19B). Some dislocations reduce in the open mouth position. With severe disease, the displaced meniscus may become distorted or misshapen. The condyle may also show osteophytic changes.

MISCELLANEOUS BONE DISORDERS

A normal bone marrow signal varies with age, depending on the proportion of red (hematopoietic) and yellow (fatty) marrow present. On T1-weighted images, red marrow is intermediate to low in signal intensity, and yellow marrow has a high signal intensity. New-

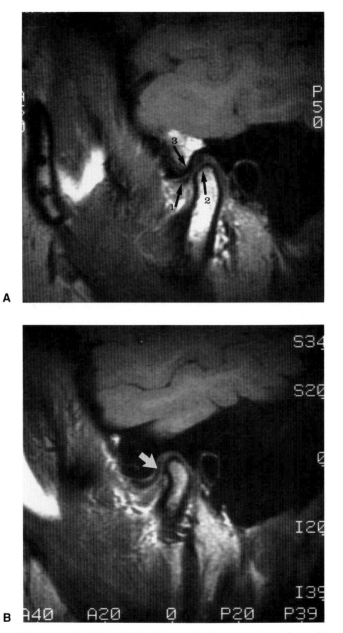

FIG. 19. TMJ. An oblique sagittal T1-weighted image in the closed mouth position. **A:** Normal TMJ. The bow-tie-shaped low-signal-intensity meniscus (*1*) has its thin intermediate zone interposed between the mandibular condyle (*2*) and the articular eminence (*3*) of the temporal zone. **B:** Meniscal dislocation. The meniscus is displaced anterior to the mandibular condyle with mild distortion of the posterior band (*arrow*).

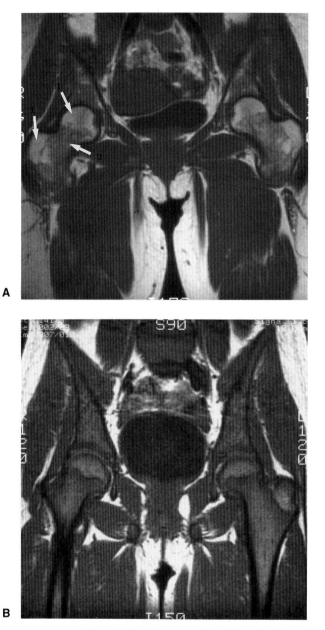

FIG. 20. Bone marrow in coronal T1-weighted images of the hips. **A:** Normal hyperintense yellow marrow (*1*) is seen in the femoral heads and greater trochanters. Residual intermediate-signal-intensity red marrow (*2*) is present in the femoral necks. **B:** Intermediate-signal-intensity red marrow fills the pelvis and hips in this patient with sickle cell anemia. Conversion to yellow matter has not occurred.

borns have mostly red marrow. Most red marrow spaces are progressively converted to yellow marrow by adulthood. In hemolytic anemias, the red marrow spaces are expanded because of increased hematopoiesis, and conversion to yellow marrow may not occur (Fig. 20).

Traumatic, inflammatory, and neoplastic processes of bone also cause a decreased marrow signal intensity on T1-weighted images. This is caused by an increased water content (edema or increased cellularity), rather than by expansion of red marrow spaces. In addition to the clinical history, other factors that sug-

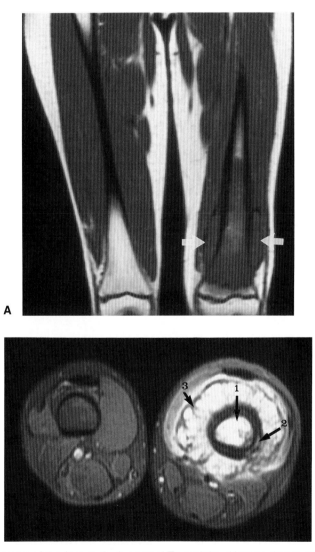

FIG. 21. Osteosarcoma of the femur. **A:** A coronal T1-weighted image demonstrates an abnormally low signal intensity in the distal diaphysis and metaphysis on the left. Periosteal elevation is also seen (*arrows*). **B:** An axial T2-weighted fat-saturated image shows hyperintense marrow (*1*), a high signal intensity within the normally hypointense bony cortex (*2*), and a hyperintense "star-burst" periosteal elevation (*3*).

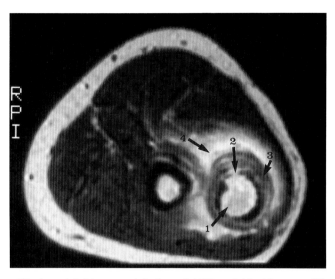

FIG. 22. Osteomyelitis (coccidioidomycosis). An axial T2-weighted image of the forearm demonstrates an abnormal ulna. A hyperintense marrow signal (*1*), high signal within the cortex (*2*), and periosteal elevation (*3*) are present, with surrounding soft tissue edema (*4*). The aggressive appearance of this lesion might suggest a malignant tumor.

gest a tumor, inflammation, or trauma are focal involvement, associated periosteal elevation, adjacent soft tissue swelling, and an abnormally high signal intensity in the bony cortex. These findings are often best seen as an increased signal intensity on fat-saturated T2-weighted sequences (Fig. 21). Differentiation of a tumor from infection or trauma can be difficult by MRI (Fig. 22). Furthermore, benign lesions cannot be differentiated from malignant tumors by MRI with certainty. In general, the more aggressive the appearance is, the more likely it is to be a malignant tumor. Fractures can usually be differentiated by a well-defined fracture line, often with displaced fragments (Fig. 23).

A relatively common disorder, AVN often involves the hips; MRI is the most sensitive and specific method for the diagnosis of AVN. Risk factors include corticosteroid use and sickle cell anemia. Hip involvement is often bilateral. The "double-line" sign often seen with

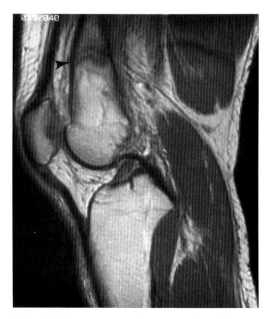

FIG. 23. Fracture. A sagittal proton density image demonstrates a transverse fracture through the femoral metaphysis (*arrow*).

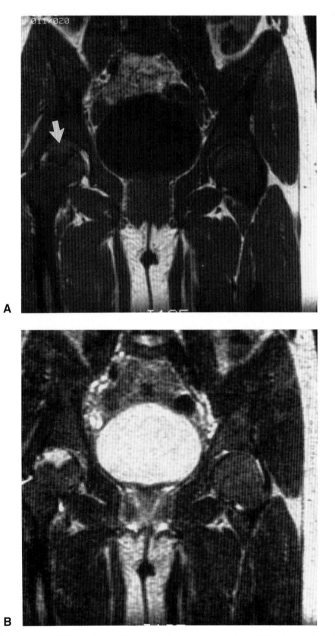

FIG. 24. AVN. **A:** A coronal T1-weighted image shows expansion of the low-signal-intensity red marrow space in sickle cell anemia; AVN is present in the right femoral head (*arrow*) surrounded by a serpiginous hypointense rim. **B:** A T2-weighted image shows marked hyperintensity in the lesion.

MRI on T2-weighted images is virtually diagnostic. It consists of a well-defined serpentine low-signal-intensity rim geographically surrounding a high-signal-intensity center (Fig. 24). Usually, AVN is homogeneously low in signal intensity on T1 weighting. The findings of AVN can be variable, however, being homogeneously low in signal intensity on T2 or bright on T1; it may be diffuse as opposed to geographic. In late stages, femoral head deformity and degenerative arthritis may be present; MRI is the modality of choice in evaluating the early changes of AVN.

SOFT TISSUE ABNORMALITIES

Most musculoskeletal soft tissue abnormalities are benign. Depending on the lesion, detection by MRI is usually based on the increased content of water, fat, hemorrhage, or fibrosis. Obtaining both a T1- and T2-weighted sequence (usually in the axial plane) is essential to determine the lesion's composition. Fat saturation can be helpful on T2 weighting to increase the sensitivity of detection. It also confirms the presence of fat, a differentiation from high-signal-intensity hemorrhage. Coro-

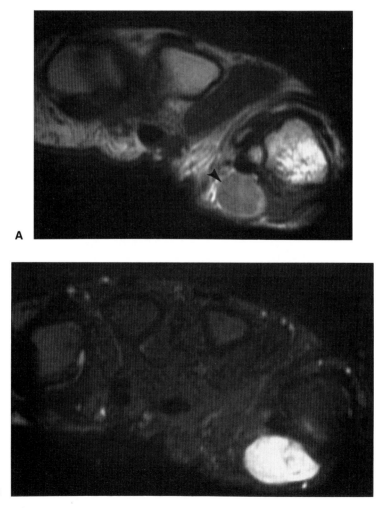

FIG. 25. Neurofibroma. **A:** An axial T1-weighted image demonstrates an intermediate-signal-intensity mass (*arrow*) in the thenar eminence. **B:** A T2-weighted fat-saturated image shows a hyperintense signal with mild internal heterogeneity.

nal and sagittal imaging planes are often useful to define the extent of tumor further.

Most solid lesions are low to intermediate in signal intensity (similar to muscle) on T1 and hyperintense on T2 weighting (Fig. 25). Exceptions to this rule include lipomas, which are isointense to subcutaneous fat; fibrosis, which has a low signal intensity on both T1 and T2 weighting; and foreign bodies, which are variable but often have a low signal intensity. Cysts are generally isointense with water (low T1-weighted and high T2-weighted signal, Fig. 26). They can usually be differentiated from a solid lesion by their uniform appearance and markedly hyperintense signal on T2. For difficult cases, gadolinium administration can be helpful. Solid lesions often enhance (except foreign bodies), whereas cysts do not.

Well-circumscribed homogeneous soft tissue lesions are most likely benign. Some benign lesions, however, are heterogeneous. These include hematomas and hemangiomas. The signal characteristics of a hematoma depend on its age (see Chapter 1). Multiple stages of blood products are often present within a single hematoma, which accounts for its signal heterogeneity (Fig. 27). Adjacent edema, which is hyperintense on T2 weighting, can make the surrounding margins appear poorly defined and give a hematoma an aggressive appearance.

Hemangiomas are benign vascular tumors. They are typically slightly hyperintense to muscle on T1 and markedly hyperintense on T2 weighting. Serpiginous vascular structures may be present within them. Often, the lesions contain fatty elements and fibrous stands that contribute to their heterogeneity in signal intensity and appearance (Fig. 28).

Malignant soft tissue sarcomas frequently have an aggressive appearance. They tend to have poorly defined borders, may invade adjacent structures, and cross fascial planes. Signal heterogeneity is also common, which is often secondary to necrosis and hemorrhage (Fig. 29). Postoperatively or postradiation therapy, tumor recurrence can be detected on T2-weighted images by the presence of high-signal-intensity tissue at the operative site. Postoperative fibrosis is low in signal intensity. To exclude tumor recurrence by signal characteristics alone can be difficult. This is because posttreatment edema (bright on T2) may persist for weeks or months. The T1 appearance may be useful. For soft tissue sarcomas, a muscular texture seen in the postoperative site is evidence for a lack of tumor recurrence. Low-signal-intensity tissue without the appearance of muscular texture on T1 may indicate recurrent tumor.

CONGENITAL

Congenital hip dislocation is well demonstrated by MRI. In addition to the femoral head position, associated deformity of the femoral head and acetabulum can be determined (Fig. 30).

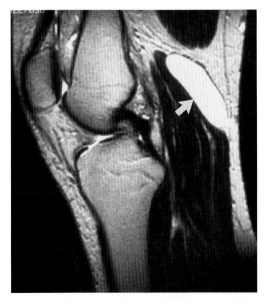

FIG. 26. Baker (popliteal) cyst. A sagittal T2-weighted image demonstrates an oval, well-circumscribed, homogeneous, and markedly hyperintense mass (*arrow*) in the popliteal fossa.

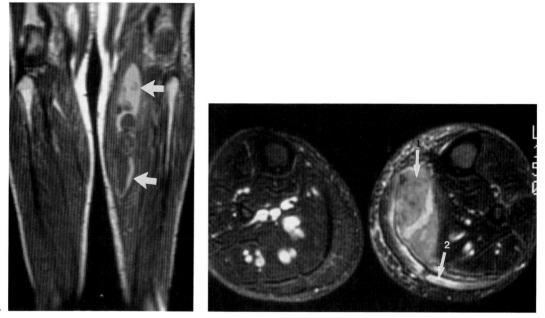

FIG. 27. Hematoma (traumatic). **A:** A coronal T1-weighted image demonstrates a calf mass (*arrows*) with components of variable signal intensity, which represent multiple blood products. **B:** An axial T2-weighted fat-saturated image demonstrates a heterogeneous hematoma (*1*) with surrounding hyper-intense edema (*2*). The presence of edema may suggest an aggressive process.

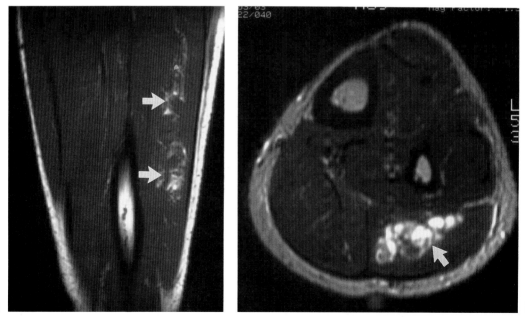

FIG. 28. Soft tissue hemangioma. **A:** A coronal T1-weighted image demonstrates increased fatty el-ements (*arrows*) within the lateral gastrocnemius muscle. **B:** An axial T2-weighted image shows the heterogeneous mass (*arrow*) containing fluid components and fibrous (low signal intensity) septa.

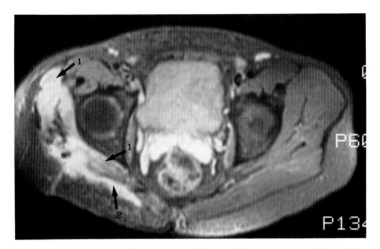

FIG. 29. Soft tissue sarcoma. An axial T2-weighted image demonstrates a hyperintense signal within the gluteus muscles on the right (*1*), extending into the tensor fascia lata anteriorly. Surrounding edema (*2*) is seen deep to the subcutaneous fat.

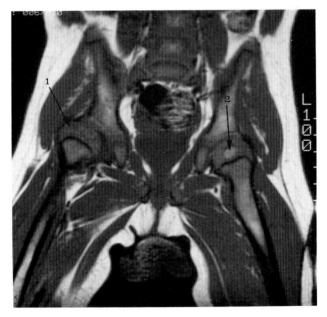

FIG. 30. Congenital hip dislocation. A coronal T1-weighted image demonstrates superior displacement of the right femoral head (*1*) and a shallow acetabular roof. Maturation of the femoral epiphysis is also delayed on the right compared with the left (*2*).

BIBLIOGRAPHY

Books

1. Stoller DW. *Magnetic resonance imaging in orthopaedics and sports medicine.* Philadelphia: JB Lippincott; 1993.
2. Zlatkin MB. *MRI of the shoulder.* New York: Raven Press;1991.
3. Higgins CB, Hricak H, Helms CA. *Magnetic imaging of the body.* New York: Raven Press; 1992.

Journals

1. Yao L, Lee JK. Occult interosseous fracture: detection with MR imaging. *Radiology* 1988;167:749–751.
2. Mink JH, Deutsch AL. Occult cartilage and bone injuries of the knee: detection, classification, and assessment with MR imaging. *Radiology* 1989;170:823–829.
3. DeSmet AA, Fisher DR, Graf BK, Lange RH. Osteochondritis desiccans of the knee: value of MR imaging in determining lesion stability and the presence of articular cartilage defects. *AJR Am J Roentgenol* 1990;155:549–553.
4. Chan WP, Lang P, Stevens MP, et al. Osteoarthritis of the knee: comparison of radiography, CT, and MR imaging to assess extent and severity. *AJR Am J Roentgenol* 1991;157:799–806.
5. Mink JH, Levy T, Crues JV III. Tears of the anterior cruciate ligament and menisci of the knee: MR imaging evaluation. *Radiology* 1988;167:769–774.
6. Lee JK, Yao L, Phelps CT, Wirth CR, Czajka J, Lozeman J. Anterior cruciate ligament tears: MR imaging compared with arthroscopy and clinical tests. *Radiology* 1988;166:861–864.
7. Burk DL, Mitchell DG, Rifkin MD, Vinitski S. Recent advances in magnetic resonance imaging of the knee. *Radiol Clin North Am* 1990;28:379–393.
8. Stoller DW, Martin C, Crues JV III, Kaplan L, Mink JH. Meniscal tears: pathologic correlation with MR imaging. *Radiology* 1987;163:731–735.
9. Crues JV III, Mink J, Levy TL, Lotysch M, Stoller DW. Meniscal tears of the knee: accuracy of MR imaging. *Radiology* 1987;164:445–448.
10. Weiss KL, Morehouse HT, Levy IM. Sagittal MR images of the knee: a low signal band parallel to the posterior cruciate ligament caused by a displaced bucket-handle tear. *AJR Am J Roentgenol* 1991;156:117–119.
11. Herman LJ, Beltran J. Pitfalls in MR imaging of the knee. *Radiology* 1988;167:775–781.
12. Seeger LL, Gold RH, Bassett LW, Ellman H. Shoulder impingement syndrome: MR findings in 53 shoulders. *AJR Am J Roentgenol* 1988;150:343–347.
13. Farley TE, Neuman CH, Steinbach LS, Jahnke AJ, Petersen SS. Full-thickness tears of the rotator cuff on the shoulder: diagnosis with MR imaging. *AJR Am J Roentgenol* 1992;158:347–351.
14. Rafil M, Firooznia H, Sherman O, et al. Rotator cuff lesions: signal patterns at MR imaging. *Radiology* 1990;177:817–823.
15. Davis SJ, Teresi LM, Bradley WG, Ressler JA, Eto RT. Effect of arm rotation on MR imaging of the rotator cuff. *Radiology* 1991;181:265–268.
16. Erickson SJ, Cox IH, Hyde JS, Carrera GF, Strandt JA, Estkowski LD. Effect of tendon orientation on MR imaging signal intensity: a manifestation of the "magic angle" phenomenon. *Radiology* 1991;181:389–392.
17. Kaplan PA, Bryans KC, Davick JP, Otte M, Stinson WW, Dussault RG. MR imaging of the shoulder: variants and pitfalls. *Radiology* 1992;184:519–524.
18. Neumann CH, Peterson SA, Jahnke AH. MR imaging of the labral-capsular complex: normal variations. *AJR Am J Roentgenol* 1991;157:1015–1021.
19. McCauley TR, Pope CF, Jokl P. Normal and abnormal glenoid labrum: assessment with multiplanar gradient-echo MR imaging. *Radiology* 1992;183:35–37.
20. Flannigan B, Kursunoglu-Brahmes, S, Snyder S, Karzel R, Del Pizzo W, Resnick D. MR arthrography of the shoulder: comparison with conventional MR imaging. *AJR Am J Roentgenol* 1990;155:829–832.
21. Middleton WD, Kneeland JB, Kellman GM, et al. MR imaging of the carpal tunnel: normal anatomy and preliminary findings in the carpal tunnel syndrome. *AJR Am J Roentgenol* 1987;148:307–316.
22. Zlatkin MB, Chao PC, Osterman AL, Schnall MD, Dalinka MK, Kressel HY. Chronic wrist pain: evaluation with high-resolution MR imaging. *Radiology* 1989;173:723–729.
23. Reinus WR, Conway WF, Totty WG, et al. Carpal avascular necrosis: MR imaging. *Radiology* 1986; 160:689–693.
24. Helms CA, Kabon LB, McNeill C, Dodson T. Temporomandibular joint: morphology and signal intensity characteristics of the disk at MR imaging. *Radiology* 1989;172:817–820.
25. Moore SG, Dawson KL. Red and yellow marrow in the femur: age related changes in appearance at MR imaging. *Radiology* 1990;175:219–223.
26. Rao VM, Fishman M, Mitchell DG, et al. Painful sickle cell crisis: bone marrow patterns observed with MR imaging. *Radiology* 1986;161:211–215.
27. Ruzal-Shapiro C, Berdon WE, Cohen MD, Abramson SJ. MR imaging of diffuse bone marrow replacement in pediatric patients with cancer. *Radiology* 1991; 181:587–589.
28. Sundaram M, McLeod RA. MR imaging of tumor and tumorlike lesions of bone and soft tissue. *AJR Am J Roentgenol* 1990;155:817–824.
29. Deutsch AL, Mink JH, Waxman AD. Occult fractures of the proximal femur: MR imaging. *Radiology* 1989;170:113–116.
30. Mitchell DG, Rao VM, Dalinka MK, et al. Femoral head avascular necrosis: correlation of MR imaging, radiographic staging, radionuclide imaging and clinical findings. *Radiology* 1987;162:709–715.
31. Dooms CG, Hricak H, Solitto RA, Higgins CB. Lipomatous tumors and tumors with fatty component: MR imaging potential and comparison of MR and CT results. *Radiology* 1985;157:479–483.

32. Rubin JI, Gomori JM, Grossman RI, Gefter WB, Kressel HY. High field MR imaging of extracranial hematomas. *AJR Am J Roentgenol* 1987;148:813–817.

33. Cohen EK, Kressel HY, Perosio T, et al. MR imaging of soft-tissue hemangiomas: correlation with pathologic findings. *AJR Am J Roentgenol* 1988;150:1079–1081.

34. Demas BE, Heelan RT, Lane J, Marcove R, Hajdu S, Brennan MF. Soft-tissue sarcomas of the extremities: comparison of MR and CT in determining the extent of disease. *AJR Am J Roentgenol* 1988;150:615–620.

35. Biondetti PR, Ehman, RL. Soft-tissue sarcomas: use of textural patterns in skeletal muscle as a diagnostic feature in postoperative MRI. *Radiology* 1992; 183:845–848.

Glossary

B_0 The static magnetic field (a vector quantity).

Cine A sequence consisting of multiple images taken at the same spatial location but in different equally spaced intervals (usually 16) during the cardiac cycle. When seen in rapid succession, each location is viewed as a movie.

Echo time (TE) The time selected to wait after the initiation of TR to receive the radiofrequency "echo" from the patient.

Echo train The number of phase-encoding steps that are simultaneously acquired in fast spin–echo sequences.

Fast spin–echo *(FSE)* A spin–echo sequence that results in decreased scanning time by acquiring multiple phase-encoding steps simultaneously.

Fat saturation (fat-sat) A sequence that decreases the signal contribution from fat in an image. This is accomplished with a special excitation pulse that is centered on the Larmor frequency of fat.

Field of view (FOV) The width in centimeters of a square field that has been prescribed to scan a region of interest (i.e., body part). The pixels are then assigned by the system software to fill the square field exactly.

Flip angle The angle (in degrees) that the proton axis is shifted from B_0 during the excitation pulse (beginning of the repetition time [TR]).

Flow compensation (FC) A complex gradient added to an imaging sequence to normalize the velocity effects of flow. This results in a more homogeneous signal from the fluid in motion.

Gating A method that triggers the initiation of the TR with the patient's heart beat (QRS complex). Peripheral gating (PG) uses the pulsatility at a finger or toe for triggering. Electrocardiographic gating (ECG) uses the electrical activity of the heart for initiating each TR. The TR of a gated sequence is in part determined by the patient's heart rate.

Gradient-recalled echo (GRE, Grass) A technique that reduces the imaging time by eliminating the 180° refocusing pulse required in spin–echo imaging. Each acquisition yields a single slice.

Inversion recovery (STIR) A sequence that uses the difference in relaxation times between fat and water to null the signal contribution of fat on an image.

Larmor frequency The characteristic frequency in which a molecule's protons (e.g., fat and water) precess in the external magnetic field (B_0).

Matrix The number of frequency- and phase-encoding steps prescribed (usually 128, 192, or 256). This determines the number and size of the pixels present in the FOV.

Multiplanar GRE (MPGR) A GRE sequence in which sampling for multiple slices is obtained during a single TR.

NEX The number of excitations performed and averaged for each phase-encoding step.

No phase wrap (NP) An imaging option that doubles the number of phase-encoding steps and then discards the added steps at the edges of the FOV. This prevents anatomy outside the FOV from contributing to the image signal inside the FOV.

Phase encoding The process whereby pixel localization along one matrix axis is determined by a series of excitation steps (each taking time

TR). Each step is encoded by a slight proton spin phase change.

Repetition time (TR)   The time that elapses between two consecutive excitation pulses (phase encoding steps).

Spatial saturation (SAT)   A radiofrequency pulse applied to anatomy outside the FOV. This reduces any artifact within the FOV that would otherwise occur from motion outside the FOV.

Spin echo   A sequence that adds a 180° pulse at one-half the TE to refocus the precessing protons at time TE. This helps maximize the signal and minimize artifacts that result from magnetic field inhomogeneities.

Spoiled GRE (SPGR)   A GRE sequence in which a "spoiler" pulse is applied just prior to the initiation of TR to eliminate residual transverse magnetization. This results in the appearance of T1 weighting and an improved signal-to-noise ratio (SNR).

Three-dimensional acquisition   Image acquisition is performed as a volume rather than as a series of planar slices.

Time of flight (TOF)   A term used to describe the increase in intravascular signal seen with blood flow that is perpendicular to the plane of the slice. This effect results from blood moving into the imaging plane after receiving its excitation outside the imaging plane.

T1   (spin-lattice relaxation) A time that corresponds to the vector realignment (along the z-axis) of the excited protons to the applied magnetic field, B_0. T1 effects predominate when a short TR and a short TE are prescribed (T1 weighting).

T2   (spin-spin relaxation) A time that corresponds to the dispersion of the vector alignment (into the xy-plane) of excited protons because of differences in precession rates. T2 effects predominate when a long TR and a long TE are prescribed (T2 weighting).

Appendix

Imaging Protocols

HEAD/NECK

SCREENING BRAIN

PLANE	PULSE	TE	TE2	TR	ET	FLIP	FOV	SLICE	GAP	#SLICES	MATRIX	NEX	FREQ	OPTIONS	TIME (MIN)
1 SAG	SE	16		651			22	5	1.5	15	192	1	SI	S(I) NP	2:23
2 AX	FSE	85		3200	8		20-22	5	2.5	18	256	1	AP	S(I)	1:23
3 AX	FSE	17		2000	4		20-22	5	2.5	18	256	1	AP	S(I)	1:40
4 AX	SE	16		651			20-22	5	2.5	18	192	2	AP	NONE	3:56
5 AX	SE	30	70	2300			20-22	5	2.5	18	192	1	AP	FC S(I) VB	7:22

FOR CORONAL PLANE USE AXIAL PARAMETERS

PEDIATRIC BRAIN (>12 MONTHS)

PLANE	PULSE	TE	TE2	TR	ET	FLIP	FOV	SLICE	GAP	#SLICES	MATRIX	NEX	FREQ	OPTIONS	TIME (MIN)
1 SAG	SE	16		651			18-20	5	1.5	15	192	1	SI	S(I) NP	2:05
2 AX	SE	30	100	2500			18-20	5	2.5	36-40	192	1	AP	FC S(I) VB	8:00
3 AX	SE	16		600			18-20	5	2.5	18-20	192	2	AP	NONE	3:55

FOR CORONAL PLANE USE AXIAL PARAMETERS

INFANT BRAIN (<12 MONTHS)

PLANE	PULSE	TE	TE2	TR	ET	FLIP	FOV	SLICE	GAP	#SLICES	MATRIX	NEX	FREQ	OPTIONS	TIME (MIN)
1 SAG	SE	15		600			18	4	1	14	192	2	SI	S(I) NP	3:55
2 AX	SE	60	120	3000			18	4-5	1.5-2	36	192	1	AP	FC S(I) VB	9:36
3 AX	SE	15		600			18	4-5	1.5-2	18	192	2	AP	NONE	3:55

FOR CORONAL PLANE USE AXIAL PARAMETERS

SEIZURE

PLANE	PULSE	TE	TE2	TR	ET	FLIP	FOV	SLICE	GAP	#SLICES	MATRIX	NEX	FREQ	OPTIONS	TIME (MIN)
1 SAG	SE	16		651			22	5	1.5	15	192	1	SI	S(I) NP	2:23
2 AX	FSE	85		3200			20-22	5	2.5	18	256	1	AP	S(I)	1:23
3 AX	FSE	17		2000			20-22	5	2.5	18	256	1	AP	S(I)	1:40
4 COR	SE	30	70	GATED (3 RR)		20	5	2.5	36	192	1	SI	FC S(I) VB		

PITUITARY

PLANE	PULSE	TE	TE2	TR	ET	FLIP	FOV	SLICE	GAP	#SLICES	MATRIX	NEX	FREQ	OPTIONS	TIME (MIN)
1 SAG	SE	15		525			19	3	0.5	12	192	4	SI	S(I) NP	6:45
2 AX	FSE	85		3200			20-22	5	2.5	18	256	1	AP	S(I)	1:23
3 AX	FSE	17		2000			20-22	5	2.5	18	256	1	SI	S(I)	1:40
4 COR	SE	15		525			19	3	0.5	12	192	4	SI	S(I)	6:45

MULTIPLE SCLEROSIS

PLANE	PULSE	TE	TE2	TR	ET	FLIP	FOV	SLICE	GAP	#SLICES	MATRIX	NEX	FREQ	OPTIONS	TIME (MIN)
1 SAG	FSE	17	107	3000	8		22	4	2	30	192	1	SI	S(I) NP FSE2	4:11
2 AX	SE	30	70	2300			20-22	5	2.5	18	192	1	AP	FC S(I) VB	7:22
3 AX	SE	16		651			20-22	5	2.5	18	192	2	AP	NONE	3:56

INTERNAL AUDITORY CANALS

PLANE	PULSE	TE	TE2	TR	ET	FLIP	FOV	SLICE	GAP	#SLICES	MATRIX	NEX	FREQ	OPTIONS	TIME (MIN)
1 SAG	SE	16		651			22	5	1.5	15	192	1	SI	S(I) NP	2:23
2 AX	FSE	85		3200			20-22	5	2.5	18	256	1	AP	S(I)	1:23
3 AX	FSE	17		2000			20-22	5	2.5	18	256	1	AP	S(I)	1:40
4 AX	SE	MIN		600			19	3	0.5	10	192	4	AP	S(S,I) FC	7:40
5 AX	SE	MIN		600			19	3	0.5	10	192	4	AP	S(S,I) FC	7:40

WITH GAD

HEAD/NECK (contd.)
ORBITS

PLANE	PULSE	TE	TE2	TR	ET	FLIP	FOV	SLICE	GAP	#SLICES	MATRIX	NEX	FREQ	OPTIONS	TIME (MIN)
1 SAG	SE	16		651			22	5	1.5	15	192	1	SI	S(I) NP	2:23
2 AX	FSE	85		3200	8		20-22	5	2.5	18	256	1	AP	S(I)	1:23
3 AX	FSE	17		2000	4		20-22	5	2.5	18	256	1	AP	S(I)	1:40
4 COR	SE	15		651			16	3	1	12	192	4	SI	S(FAT) NP	7:50
5 COR	SE	15		651			16	3	1	12	192	4	SI	S(FAT) NP	7:50

WITH GAD: FOR AXIAL T1 USE CORONAL PARAMETERS

POSTERIOR FOSSA

PLANE	PULSE	TE	TE2	TR	ET	FLIP	FOV	SLICE	GAP	#SLICES	MATRIX	NEX	FREQ	OPTIONS	TIME (MIN)
1 SAG	SE	16		651			22	5	1.5	15	192	1	SI	S(I) NP	2:25
2 AX	FSE	85		3200	8		20-22	5	2.5	18	256	1	AP	S(I)	1:23
3 AX	FSE	17		2000	4		20-22	5	2.5	18	256	1	AP	S(I)	1:40
4 AX	SE	29		700			20-22	4	1	12	192	2	AP	S(SI) FC	7:40

MR ANGIO 3D TOF

PLANE	PULSE	TE	TE2	TR	ET	FLIP	FOV	SLICE	GAP	#SLICES	MATRIX	NEX	FREQ	OPTIONS	TIME (MIN)
1 AX	SPGR	4.5		50		20	19	1.0	0	80	192	1	AP	S(SAPRL) FC	10:00

CIRCLE OF WILLIS (VOLUME ACQUISITION)

MR ANGIO PHASE CONTRAST

PLANE	PULSE	TE	TE2	TR	ET	FLIP	FOV	SLICE	GAP	#SLICES	MATRIX	NEX	FREQ	OPTIONS	TIME (MIN)
1 AX	GRE	5		50		20	14	1.0	0	28	128	1	AP	PG GRX	9:00

CIRCLE OF WILLIS (VOLUME ACQUISITION)

MR ANGIO 2D TOF

PLANE	PULSE	TE	TE2	TR	ET	FLIP	FOV	SLICE	GAP	#SLICES	MATRIX	NEX	FREQ	OPTIONS	TIME (MIN)
1 AX	SPGR	MIN		45		60	18	1.5	0	64	128	1	AP	S(I) FC GRX	9:10

CAROTIDS (NECK COIL)

BRAIN VENOGRAM

PLANE	PULSE	TE	TE2	TR	ET	FLIP	FOV	SLICE	GAP	#SLICES	MATRIX	NEX	FREQ	OPTIONS	TIME (MIN)
1 COR	SPGR	MIN		45		40	20	1.5	0	128	128	1	SI	S(I) FC	9:00

NASOPHARYNX

PLANE	PULSE	TE	TE2	TR	ET	FLIP	FOV	SLICE	GAP	#SLICES	MATRIX	NEX	FREQ	OPTIONS	TIME (MIN)
1 SAG	SE	16		651			24	5	1.5	15	192	1	SI	S(I) NP	2:25
2 AX	FSE	55		3600	8		20	5	1.5	17	256	1	AP	S(SI,FAT)	1:23
3 AX	SE	15		400			20	5	1.5	18	192	2	AP	S(SI)	4:45
4 COR	SE	15		650			20	5	1.5	15	192	2	SI	S(SI) NP	5:45

NECK

PLANE	PULSE	TE	TE2	TR	ET	FLIP	FOV	SLICE	GAP	#SLICES	MATRIX	NEX	FREQ	OPTIONS	TIME (MIN)
1 COR	SE	15		300			24	5	2.5	12	192	2	SI	S(SI) NP	3:58
2 AX	FSE	55		3600	8		20	5	2.5	17	256	1	AP	S(SI,FAT)	1:23
3 AX	SE	15		300			20	5	2.5	18	128	4	AP	S(SI)	7:30

SPINE
CERVICAL DISC

PLANE	PULSE	TE	TE2	TR	ET	FLIP	FOV	SLICE	GAP	#SLICES	MATRIX	NEX	FREQ	OPTIONS	TIME (MIN)
1 SAG	SE	15		550			24	3	1	12	192	4	SI	S(ASI) NP	7:00
2 SAG	FSE	85		2200	8		24	3	1	9	256	2	AP	S(APSI) NP PG	2:30
3 AX	MPGR	14		700		20	24	3	1	26	192	2	RL	S(API) NP FC	9:20

	PLANE	PULSE	TE	TE2	ET	TR	FLIP	FOV	SLICE	GAP	#SLICES	MATRIX	NEX	FREQ	OPTIONS	TIME (MIN)
SPINE (contd.)																
CERVICAL CORD																
	1 SAG	SE	15			550		24	3	1	12	192	4	SI	S(ASI) NP	7:00
	2 SAG	FSE	85			2200		24	3	1	9	256	2	AP	S(APSI) NP PG	2:30
	3 AX	SE	15			800		24	3	1	20	192	2	RL	S(API) NP	6:30
	4 SAG	SE	30	70		GATED		22	3	1.5	22	192	1	S1	NP PG FC	
THORACIC DISC AND CORD																
	1 SAG	SE	15			524		30	3	1	12	192	4	SI	S(API)	6:45
	2 SAG	FSE	102			GATED		30	3	1	6-9	256	2	AP	S(API) PG NP	
	3 AX	SE	15			800		24	3	1	20	192	2	RL	S(API) NP	6:30
	4 SAG	VE/MPGR	15	31		600	20	30	4	0	11	192	4	SI	S(I)	8:00
LUMBAR DISC																
	1 SAG	SE	15			524		24	3	1	12	192	4	SI	S(AP)	7:28
	2 SAG	FSE	17	102	8	2000		24	4	1	22	256	2	SI	S(AP)	4:11
	3 AX	FSE	17	102	8	4000		18	5	1	40	256	1	RL	S(AP)	4:11
LUMBAR DISC POST-OP																
	1 SAG	SE	15			524		30	3	1	12	192	4	SI	S(API)	6:45
	2 AX	SE	15			400		18	5	1	20	192	2	AP	S(AP)	5:25
	REPEAT BOTH SEQUENCES POST GAD															
LUMBAR SPINE, PEDI																
	1 SAG	SE	15			524		18-24	3	1	12	192	4	SI	S(AP) NP	7:28
	2 AX	SE	15			400		16-18	3	1.5	20	192	4	AP	S(AP) NP	7:45
BODY																
BRACHIAL PLEXUS																
	1 COR	SE	15			300		30	5	2.5	12	192	2	SI	S(SI) NP	3:58
	2 AX	SE	15	60		2000		30	5	2.5	40	128	2	RL	S(SI) NP RC	9:30
	3 AX	SE	15			300		30	5	2.5	20	128	4	RL	S(SI) NP	9:00
	4 SAG	SE	15			500		24	5	2.5	20	128	2	SI	S(SI) NP	5:45
CHEST																
	1 COR	SE	15			GATED (1 RR)	32	7	3		128	2	SI	S(SI) ECG RC		
	2 AX	SE	15	60		GATED (3RR)	30-32	7	3		128	2	RL	S(SI) ECG RC		
	3 AX	SE	15			GATED (1RR)	30-32	7	3		128	4	RL	S(SI) ECG RC		
	FOR PEDI USE HEAD COIL AND SMALLER FOV															
HEART																
	1 AX	CINE	13			25	45	30-32	5-10	0	9	128	2	RL	S(SI) RC FC	10:00
	DO CHEST STUDY AND ADD THIS SEQUENCE. FOR PEDI USE HEAD COIL AND SMALLER FOV															

BODY (contd.)

ABDOMEN

PLANE	PULSE	TE	TE2	TR	ET	FLIP	FOV	SLICE	GAP	#SLICES	MATRIX	NEX	FREQ	OPTIONS	TIME (MIN)
1 COR	SE	15		300			28-36	5-7	2.5-3	12	128	2	SI	S(SI) RC NP	3:45
2 AX	SE	20	70	2500			28-36	5-7	2.5-3	48	128	2	RL	S(SI) RC NP	12:00
3 AX	SE	15		300			28-36	5-7	2.5-3	24	128	4	RL	S(SI) RC NP	10:17
4 AX	GRE	13		22		30	28-36	7.5-10	0	24	128	2	RL	FC NP	2:56
3 SLICES PER BREATH HOLD															
5 AX	FSE	85		4500	8		28-32	5-7	2.5-3	24	192	4	RL	S(SI,FAT) NP	7:12
FOR PEDI USE HEAD COIL AND SMALLER FOV															

PELVIS

PLANE	PULSE	TE	TE2	TR	ET	FLIP	FOV	SLICE	GAP	#SLICES	MATRIX	NEX	FREQ	OPTIONS	TIME (MIN)
1 COR	SE	15		300			28-36	5-7	2.5-3	12	128	2	SI	S(SI) NP	5:45
2 AX	FSE	85	107	4000	8		28-36	5	2.5	18	192	2	RL	S(SI) NP	3:12
3 AX	SE	15		300			28-36	5	2.5	18	128	4	RL	S(SI) NP	7:45
4 SAG	FSE	85		4000	8		28-30	5	2.5	18	192	2	SI	S(SI) NP	6:13
5 AX	GRE	13		22		30	28-36	7.5-10	0	24	128	2	RL	FC NP	2:56

EXTREMITY/ORTHO

HIPS

PLANE	PULSE	TE	TE2	TR	ET	FLIP	FOV	SLICE	GAP	#SLICES	MATRIX	NEX	FREQ	OPTIONS	TIME (MIN)
1 AX	MPGR	15		451		20	28-36	5	2.5	16	192	2	RL	FC	3:00
2 COR	FSE	17	107	3800	8		28-36	3	1.5	40	192	2	SI	S(SI) NP	4:25
3 COR	SE	15		600			28-36	3	1.5	20	128	2	SI	S(SI) NP	6:30

KNEE

PLANE	PULSE	TE	TE2	TR	ET	FLIP	FOV	SLICE	GAP	#SLICES	MATRIX	NEX	FREQ	OPTIONS	TIME (MIN)
1 AX	MPGR	18		600		20	17	5	1	15	128	1	RL	S(SI) FC	1:35
2 SAG	FSE	17	107	4000	8		18	3	1.5	36	256	1	SI	S(SI)	4:11
3 OBL RAD	MPGR	20		775		25	17	5	1	26	192	2	OBL	NP GRX	6:55
4 OBL SAG	FSE	100		2200	8		17	3	0.5	10	192	2	OBL	NP GRX	2:10
5 COR	SE	15		600			18	5	1	15	192	2	SI	S(I) NP	4:30

WRIST

PLANE	PULSE	TE	TE2	TR	ET	FLIP	FOV	SLICE	GAP	#SLICES	MATRIX	NEX	FREQ	OPTIONS	TIME (MIN)
1 AX	SE	15		500			48	4	2	15	192	1	RL	NONE	1:35
2 COR	SE	20		400			8	4	2	9	128	4	SI	S(SI) NP	4:11
3 COR	SE	20	80	2000			8	4	2	18	128	2	SI	S(SI) NP	7:40
4 COR	MPGR	21		400		10	8	4	2	9	128	4	SI	S(SI) NP FC	5:45
FOR AXIAL PLANE USE CORONAL PARAMETERS															

TMJ

PLANE	PULSE	TE	TE2	TR	ET	FLIP	FOV	SLICE	GAP	#SLICES	MATRIX	NEX	FREQ	OPTIONS	TIME (MIN)
1 COR	SE	MIN		300			14	4	1	9	128	2	SI	NP	2:25
2 SAG	SE	MIN		450			12	3	1.5	6	128	4	SI	S(I) NP	4:11
DO SAG SEQUENCE IN CLOSED AND PARTIAL OPEN POSITION															

EXTREMITY/ORTHO (contd.)

SHOULDER

PLANE	PULSE	TE	TE2	TR	ET	FLIP	FOV	SLICE	GAP	#SLICES	MATRIX	NEX	FREQ	OPTIONS	TIME (MIN)
1 AX	GRE	15		451		20	18	4	1	12	192	2	RL	FC NP	2:33
2 OBL COR	FSE	66		3000	8		13	4	1	12	192	4	OBL	S(S,FAT) NP GRX	5:30
3 OBL COR	SE	17		651			12	4	1	12	192	2	OBL	S(S) NP GRX	5:45
4 OBL SAG	SE	17		651			12	4	1	12	192	2	OBL	S(S) NP GRX	5:45

SHOULDER ARTHROGRAM

PLANE	PULSE	TE	TE2	TR	ET	FLIP	FOV	SLICE	GAP	#SLICES	MATRIX	NEX	FREQ	OPTIONS	TIME (MIN)
1 AX	GRE	15		451		20	18	4	1	12	192	2	RL	FC NP	2:33
2 AX	SE	15		600			18	3	1	14	128	4	RL	S(SI, R OR L)	4:45
3 OBL COR	SE	15		600			13	3	1	14	192	2	OBL	S(S) NP GRX	5:30
4 OBL SAG	SE	17		600			13	3	1	14	128	4	OBL	S(S) NP GRX	5:45
5 OBL SAG	FSE	17	107	3000	8		13	3	1	28	128	2	OBL	S(S) NP GRX	5:45

Index

Note: Page numbers followed by *f* indicate figures; those followed by *t* indicate tables.